Youth and Internet Pornography

This much-needed book provides an in-depth, nonjudgmental look at how consumption of Internet pornography and sexually explicit Internet material (SEIM) impacts the social, physical, emotional, and sexual development of adolescents.

Youth and Internet Pornography explores some of the most contemporary issues in this field, including deepfake technology, the long-standing conflict between legal challenges to pornography versus individual rights, and the interrelationship between adolescent use of Internet pornography and the larger culture. The text outlines how different generations interact with the Internet, as well as the related legal and ethical issues around working with these different age groups. Behun and Owens use clinical illustrations and guided practice exercises to contextualize theoretical constructs and research, providing a comprehensive guide to how those working with young people should consider the impact of Internet pornography in their day-to-day practice.

This book is essential reading for professionals and policy makers hoping to mitigate outcomes in counseling, youth and social work, and education, as well as supplementary reading for courses in human sexuality and development.

Dr. Richard Joseph Behun is Assistant Professor of Counselor Education at Millersville University. Dr. Behun is a licensed professional counselor, national certified counselor, and approved clinical supervisor. Dr. Behun conducts research and lectures in the areas of sexuality and the mandated reporting of child sexual abuse.

Dr. Eric W. Owens is Associate Professor of Counselor Education at West Chester University of Pennsylvania. Dr. Owens is a licensed professional counselor and certified school counselor and has worked in college, school, and clinical settings. Dr. Owens has authored texts and presented nationally and internationally on a host of counseling topics.

Adolescence and Society
Series Editor: John C. Coleman
Department of Education, University of Oxford

In the 20 years since it began, this series has published some of the key texts in the field of adolescent studies. The series has covered a very wide range of subjects, almost all of them being of central concern to students, researchers, and practitioners. A mark of its success is that a number of books have gone to second and third editions, illustrating its popularity and reputation.

The primary aim of the series is to make accessible to the widest possible readership important and topical evidence relating to adolescent development. Much of this material is published in relatively inaccessible professional journals, and the objective of the books has been to summarise, review and place in context current work in the field, so as to interest and engage both an undergraduate and a professional audience.

The intention of the authors is to raise the profile of adolescent studies among professionals and in institutions of higher education. By publishing relatively short, readable books on topics of current interest to do with youth and society, the series makes people more aware of the relevance of the subject of adolescence to a wide range of social concerns.

The books do not put forward any one theoretical viewpoint. The authors outline the most prominent theories in the field and include a balanced and critical assessment of each of these. Whilst some of the books may have a clinical or applied slant, the majority concentrate on normal development.

The readership rests primarily in two major areas: the undergraduate market, particularly in the fields of psychology, sociology and education; and the professional training market, with particular emphasis on social work, clinical and educational psychology, counselling, youth work, nursing and teacher training.

Also in this series

Young People and the Care Experience
Julie Shaw and Nick Frost

Youth and Internet Pornography
The Impact and Influence on Adolescent Development
Richard Joseph Behun and Eric W. Owens

For more information about this series, please visit:www.routledge.com/Adolescence-and-Society/book-series/SE0238

Youth and Internet Pornography
The Impact and Influence on Adolescent Development

**Richard Joseph Behun
and Eric W. Owens**

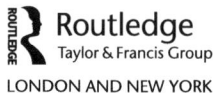

LONDON AND NEW YORK

First published 2020
by Routledge
2 Park Square, Milton Park, Abingdon, Oxon OX14 4RN

and by Routledge
52 Vanderbilt Avenue, New York, NY 10017

Routledge is an imprint of the Taylor & Francis Group, an informa business

© 2020 Richard Joseph Behun and Eric W. Owens

The right of Richard Joseph Behun and Eric W. Owens to be identified as authors of this work has been asserted by them in accordance with sections 77 and 78 of the Copyright, Designs and Patents Act 1988.

All rights reserved. No part of this book may be reprinted or reproduced or utilised in any form or by any electronic, mechanical, or other means, now known or hereafter invented, including photocopying and recording, or in any information storage or retrieval system, without permission in writing from the publishers.

Trademark notice: Product or corporate names may be trademarks or registered trademarks, and are used only for identification and explanation without intent to infringe.

British Library Cataloguing-in-Publication Data
A catalogue record for this book is available from the British Library

Library of Congress Cataloging-in-Publication Data
A catalog record for this book has been requested

ISBN: 978-1-138-39052-2 (hbk)
ISBN: 978-1-138-39053-9 (pbk)
ISBN: 978-0-429-42314-7 (ebk)

Typeset in Times New Roman
by Apex CoVantage, LLC

This text is dedicated to all of the professionals out there working to help our young people navigate the digital age. It is not easy, and it is not always fun. But it is definitely worth it, and we thank you.

Contents

Preface		x
Acknowledgments		xii

1 Strange bedfellows: adolescents and Internet pornography   1

An introduction to adolescents and SEIM 2
A few caveats 4
Terminology 5
Prevalence of adolescents' use of SEIM 7
An overview of the text 8
Conclusion 9
Summary 10
Additional resources 10
References 11

2 The digital divide: strangers in a strange land   14

Generations, defined 15
Digital immigrants and digital natives 16
Popular culture and adolescents 19
The digital native and the helping relationship 21
Conclusion 25
Summary 25
Additional resources 26
References 26

3 Thoughts and values: pornography and attitudes and beliefs   30

The Centerfold Syndrome 31
Permissive sexual attitudes 32
Gender-stereotypical sexual beliefs 34
Sexual self-development 36

From theory to practice 38
Approaches to intervention 39
Conclusion 42
Summary 42
Additional resources 43
References 43

4 From thinking to doing: the impact on behavior and sexual decision making   46

Sexual experience and casual sex 47
High risk behavior 48
Sexual aggression and victimization 49
SEIM and addiction 49
Conduct issues, substance use, and other mental health concerns 51
From theory to practice 52
Approaches to intervention 54
Conclusion 56
Summary 57
Additional resources 57
References 58

5 Thoughts of the self: pornography and adolescent self-image   61

Self-image and SEIM: understanding the relationships 62
Body image 63
Physical attractiveness 66
Genitalia and other sexual-related body parts 66
Self-esteem 68
Conclusion 69
Summary 70
Additional resources 71
References 71

6 From the self to the world: the intersection of pornography and culture   74

Age 75
Gender 76
Political ideology 77
Worldview 78
Religion 79
LGBTQ 81

Conclusion 82
Summary 84
Additional resources 85
References 85

7 Potential pitfalls: legal and ethical issues in the field   88

Ethics, law, and pornography 89
Ethical issues and obligations for helping professionals 89
Laws and legal issues and obligations for helping professionals 92
Conclusion 97
Summary 101
Additional resources 102
References 102

8 What's new? Current issues in youth and internet pornography   104

Protected speech or protecting the public: government involvement in SEIM 105
Deepfakes: artificial intelligence and pornography 109
Sexting: "send nudes" 111
Conclusion 114
Summary 114
Additional resources 115
References 115

9 Conclusion: making sense of it all   118

Technology as a cultural construct 118
Attitudes, behaviors, and self-image 119
The intersection of culture and pornography 120
Ethics and the law 121
A primer on academic research 122
Rapid evolution: the technological boom 123
Conclusion 124
Summary 124
References 125

Index   127

Preface

I'm lost. I really am. Trying to work with teenagers in this day and age? I barely knew how to set the clock on my VCR and now we have smartphones and tablets and video game systems that are on the Internet. My TV is online! I don't even know how that happened; my kids set it up. The whole world is online, and man, it's not necessarily a good thing. I mean, yeah, the world is at our fingertips, but is it always a good thing to have access to every corner of the world?

The Internet isn't going anywhere. For some, this is a welcome relief (as if there was any question that the Internet *might* be going away?). Children, adolescents, and young adults do not know a world without the Internet. There has always been access to anything you want; the entirety of the world's knowledge is available with a few keystrokes and a wireless router. But for others, the Internet could go away. Those of us who remember the buzzing sound of a dial-up connection and the words "You've got mail" could probably do without it some days.

Pornography isn't going anywhere either. There are many perspectives on pornography, and most people have some opinion about it should you ask. For some, pornography is a social catastrophe, emblematic of the crumbling of a moral and value-based society. For others, pornography is a way to explore fantasies in a healthy way or engage one's sexual partner on a different level. For still others, it may be some combination of both or something altogether different.

Finally, we have adolescents. One of the authors currently lives with an adolescent and so understands all too well the challenges that come with this stage of life. To be honest, both authors somehow successfully navigated their own adolescence but may not remember it that well anymore. Adolescence is a time of great change and plenty of dissonance. Everything seems to be changing, from one's body to one's mind.

Where these three things intersect, you'll find this text. Our purpose, which we state throughout, is not to pass any moral judgments or take a particular stance on pornography (or the Internet, for that matter). There are plenty of judgments and opinions out there for the reader to consider, many of which are available online. Instead, we hope to provide a reasoned, thoughtful consideration of adolescents and their consumption of Internet pornography. We hope we have taken as scientific an approach as possible, doing what we can to eliminate our own biases from the text and allowing the reader the opportunity to learn, evaluate, reflect, and then develop their own opinions.

Because in the end, the purpose of this text is to help. We have written this book for counselors, psychologists, social workers, health-care professionals and other human service providers who work with adolescent populations. It might also be helpful for parents or other caregivers to read to better understand the challenges facing our own kids. It's a confusing world out there, and one that isn't getting any easier. We know there is no way to make it any less confusing by writing a book, but maybe we can help some adults better understand how to work with some adolescents. If so, we have accomplished what we came here to do.

Acknowledgments

No text is ever written alone, even if there is only one author. In our case, there are two, which results in twice as many people who deserve acknowledgment. Word counts limit how many of them we can consider here, but there are many more whom we might not be able to mention.

Authoring any manuscript takes time, and time is a finite resource. The time spent researching, writing, revising, writing again – it comes at the expense of time spent in other places. Thank you to Shannon, Ryan, and Katie for your patience, especially when dad was busy in his office. Thank you to Julie and Shiloh for your unconditional love and understanding. I cherish every second we spend together, and I am so happy to be going through this life journey with you both. I would also like to acknowledge that there is no greater motivation than a mother-in-law telling you to write a book in your spare time because she thinks you have too much time on your hands.

We must also acknowledge the efforts of our research assistants who made this book far easier to write. Thank you to Karen Rossmell for her time management, organization, sense of humor, and minimal complaining during this project. Taylor Schlegel was instrumental in making this work a reality. Her efforts in organizing research, reference review, and editorial assistance was invaluable. We also must recognize the efforts of Elizabeth Gilmore and Alyssa Hyduk who also worked tirelessly to make sense of our research, review various iterations of the text, and provide feedback. While still working on their degrees, Taylor, Elizabeth, and Alyssa became part of the team. We both value you very much.

We must also thank the team at Routledge/Taylor and Francis for all of their support. They have been a wonderful organization with whom to work. Finally, we thank all of the people out there researching these topics. This is difficult work, and it is an especially challenging field to find yourself in. Thanks for all that you do.

1 Strange bedfellows

Adolescents and Internet pornography

> I struggle quite a bit in my practice today. I've been a counselor for a long time, and I think I'm quite good at the work. I've been dealing with issues related to healthy sexuality for my entire career, and I've always enjoyed my work with younger people. But as I get older, they get younger, and I feel like there's a disconnect. I mean, navigating the world of adolescent sexuality has never been easy and it is completely normal for adolescents to be working through a lot during this time of their lives. But the Internet . . . the Internet has changed the game. It seems like pornography has become such a bigger part of what these kids are bringing to counseling now.

Many who work in the helping professions (e.g., counselors, psychologists, social workers, nurses, physicians) find themselves engaged in conversations with adolescents about sexuality. This has been the case for as long as there have been helping professions. Adolescence is a time of normal curiosity and experimentation. It is a period of personal growth that can shape the life that is to follow. Adolescence is, in a word, challenging.

These trials are what often bring adolescents to counseling. Navigating the world of healthy sexual relationships can cause real distress in the lives of this population. Developing mature relationships during puberty is not easy and issues related to sexual behavior challenge even the most mature teenagers. Exploring sexual identity while existing in a world of close peer relationships and constant scrutiny can be harrowing. The challenge of adolescent sexual growth can result in mental health concerns, such as depression, anxiety, and so forth.

Of course no review of adolescent sexuality would be complete without considering how pornography has intersected with technology and how this intersection impacts adolescents. Just as sexuality has always been a pressing issue for this population, so has pornography. Those of us from older generations are familiar with the stories of teenagers who stole a copy of their fathers' *Playboy* magazine and snuck off to do anything but read the articles. But the Internet has changed how adolescents consume pornography. The ubiquity of sexually explicit Internet material (SEIM) has forever changed how we think about adolescents and pornography.

For those who help teenagers navigate these challenges, the landscape has changed. The vignette at the beginning of this chapter demonstrates this difficulty;

while this population continues to exist within their time and space, counselors, psychologists, and others may have real problems understanding what it is like to be an adolescent in the ever-expanding digital age. The Internet has changed everything, from the way we communicate to how we interact with the world. Dating apps, messaging programs, and social media have changed the game, especially for the adolescents who are native to this digital world and to the helpers who might be immigrants in this unfamiliar land. The unending supply of SEIM makes our work as helping professionals more challenging than ever.

The purpose of this book is to provide insight to the helpers who work with this population. This task can be daunting because technology is constantly changing and the research surrounding it has difficulty staying abreast. Our goal in this text is not to be all inclusive; that would likely be impossible. However, we do hope to provide the reader with an understanding of how adolescents interact with SEIM and the potential effects SEIM has on this population.

After reading this chapter you should be able to

1 Explain, in broad terms, how adolescents interact with SEIM;
2 Understand how the terms *adolescent, pornography*, and *Internet* will be used throughout this text;
3 Have an understanding of the prevalence of SEIM consumption among adolescents; and
4 Describe how the text will follow in subsequent chapters.

An introduction to adolescents and SEIM

Over the past three decades, pornography has become far more commonplace than at any other point in history (Löfgren-Mårtenson & Månsson, 2010; McNair, 2002; Paul, 2005; Peter & Valkenburg, 2007). The Internet has played a significant role in this mainstreaming of pornography, providing unequaled access to encounter, consume, create, and distribute sexually explicit content. Because the Internet is global and accessible worldwide, this phenomena is not isolated to any one country or community; data suggest adolescents across the globe are engaging with SEIM more than ever (Flood, 2007; Häggström-Nordin, Sandberg, Hanson, & Tydén, 2006; Lo & Wei, 2005; Wolak, Mitchell, & Finkelhor, 2007; Sabina, Wolak, & Finkelhor, 2008).

When compared to more traditional media (e.g., radio, print, television, movies), the Internet is a highly sexualized environment (Cooper, Boies, Maheu, & Greenfield, 1999; Peter & Valkenburg, 2006a). Research demonstrates significant increases in the number of youth who are intentionally or accidentally encountering pornographic material online (Mitchell, Wolak, & Finkelhor, 2007; Wolak et al., 2007). We can safely assume that adolescents' access to SEIM is unmatched by any other medium; the sheer amount of SEIM available and the vast diversity in content is unparalleled (Coopersmith, 2006; Mitchell, Wolak, & Finkelhor, 2007). Additionally, the risk of online bullying, sexual victimization, or harassment from others is real and pervasive.

Furthermore, the Internet is present and prioritized in the lives of many youth (Lenhart, Ling, Campbell, & Purcell, 2010; Lenhart, Purcell, Smith, & Zickur,

2010; Mitchell et al., 2007). For example, in the United States, 93% of all adolescents ages 12 to 17 use the Internet, 63% go online daily, and 36% are online several times a day (Lenhart, Purcell, et al., 2010). The *World Internet Report* surveyed 12- to 14-year-olds from 13 different countries and found that 100% of British youth, 98% of Israeli youth, 96% of Czech youth, and 95% of Canadian youth reported using the Internet regularly (Lawsky, 2008). Another survey found that 98% of youth from Spain are engaged online, with the majority using the Internet on a daily basis (Gómez, Rial, Braña, Golpe, & Varela, 2017). Given that the average American teen owns 3.5 mobile devices (Lenhart, Purcell, et al., 2010), it can be assumed that a great deal of their online activity is portable and, therefore, largely unmonitored (Roberts, Foehr, & Rideout, 2005). While the statistics available in the literature are somewhat dated, we can be sure that young people live in the digital age (see Chapter 2 for more information about these topics).

The unsurpassed access to the Internet that we see today has many positive influences. In the area of sexuality, people across the life span look online for information on sexual health and education (Barak & Fisher, 2001). Through social media sites, such as Facebook, Twitter, Instagram, and so many others, people can connect socially with people in their own communities or across the world. We seek out entertainment and news online, and we use technology to work, learn, and even shop for groceries.

However, unfettered access to the online world is not without its problems. Adolescents are most often still grappling with tasks related to executive functioning and may have difficulty prioritizing, making good decisions, and mitigating potential risks. When confronted with the vast amount of information, as well as the many risks inherent in navigating the Internet, adolescents often lack the skills necessary to do so safely and in healthy ways (Delmonico & Griffin, 2008). There is also a burgeoning body of research that has found that adolescents are increasingly struggling with compulsive Internet use (CIU) and compulsive behaviors related to Internet pornography and cybersex (Delmonico & Griffin, 2008; Lam, Peng, Mai, & Jing, 2009; Rimington & Gast, 2007; van den Eijnden, Spijkerman, Vermulst, van Rooij, & Engels, 2010; Villella et al., 2011; Rumpf et al., 2014; Kawabe, Horiuchi, Ochi, Oka, & Ueno, 2016; Gómez, Rial, Braña, Golpe, & Varela, 2017).

A review of the literature during this period indicates significant increases in the volume of research examining CIU and compulsive adolescent sexual behavior related to pornography, as well as a diversity in the areas of the world studying these phenomenon, such as China (Fu, Chan, Wong, & Yip, 2010), the Netherlands (van den Eijnden et al., 2010), the United Kingdom (Gillespie, 2008), the United States (Sussman, 2007), and Taiwan (Yen et al., 2009). Consequently, it may be inferred that the impact of Internet pornography on adolescents, including compulsive, addictive, and even criminal behavior, is a global trend not isolated to any one particular culture or region.

As Internet use increases, it is important to understand the systemic impact of SEIM on adolescents. Adolescent development, for the purposes of this book, includes the predictable and significant changes that occur across various domains: physical, emotional, cognitive, social, spiritual, and sexual. Consequently, adolescents are considered one of the most susceptible audiences to sexually explicit content.

A few caveats

While it is developmentally normal for adolescents to have sexual curiosity, the extent of easy, free, and unmonitored access to pornography on the Internet begs the question: what impact, if any, does exposure to Internet pornography have on adolescents? Our goal here is to answer this question across the various developmental domains mentioned previously.

This text explores two challenging and highly controversial topics: pornography and the impact of technology on youth. Daily headlines discuss both of these topics and most people have an opinion on each. While technology is still a developing area of study, pornography is not. Personal beliefs about sexually explicit media are often based in moral beliefs and personal experiences. While we do not discount either, it is important for a text such as this one to steer clear of the subjective and focus on the objective. While research still has its subjective elements, we have tried, as best as we can, to avoid moral judgments and focus on scientific inquiry.

Learning Activity 1.1 invites readers to explore their own opinions about the topics of technology and pornography.

Learning Activity 1.1

Exploring our opinions

Read the following case study and consider your responses to the questions that follow.

Dr. Scott is a licensed psychotherapist working in private practice. She works primarily with adolescents and their families, especially around issues related to behavioral change. She began working with a young man named Rich. Rich is a 15-year-old, straight, cisgendered male who has recently started dating and has become sexually active with his girlfriend of five weeks.

Rich's parents have "required" him to seek counseling because they found "pornography" on his laptop computer. Specifically, through a search of Rich's online browsing history, they found that he had been looking at photographs of college-aged, female cheerleaders. These photographs depicted the women fully clothed and engaged in typical activities that would be found at sporting events.

During your first sessions with Rich, he argues vehemently that he was not seeking to view pornography and was not looking at the images for the purpose of sexual arousal. "I was thinking about going out for the cheerleading team," he pleads. "My parents think I'm looking at these pictures as a way of getting off, but really I just want to understand what cheerleaders do."

Consider the following:

1 Is this pornography? Why or why not?
2 Do you believe Rich's explanation of his reason for viewing these images?
3 Are the answers to these questions important? If so, what makes them important? Why does *your* opinion as a counselor matter (consider your own biases as well as how these biases may impact your work)?

Our purpose is to highlight the direct influences pornography has on the developmental processes of children and on adolescents specifically. One challenge in a text such as this is the dearth of literature that examines the impact of pornography and SEIM on minors. While the literature is rich with studies exploring the impact on adults, children and adolescents have received far less attention, in large part due to the ethical and legal considerations involved when examining these issues. In the United States, as in many other countries, it is illegal to distribute sexually explicit material to minors or knowingly expose them to it, thereby creating significant challenges when trying to explore these topics. Asking about a teenager's illegal behavior, or helping to facilitate it, is understandably difficult.

Two issues regarding this review are worthy of note; first, we have included research in which the authors may not have examined online pornography specifically but pornography in various media. We did this with the assumption that the Internet has become a universally accepted source of information, especially for adolescents, and that exposure to pornography may be assumed to occur on the Internet as frequently, if not more frequently, than through any other medium. Also, a book that examines these issues could take many directions; however, the current body of research provided the parameters for this text and emphasis has been placed on research that examines nonclinical and noncompulsive Internet pornography exposure.

Terminology

Before moving forward, it is important to understand the terminology used throughout this text. While many terms will be specific to the topics in each chapter, some definitions are warranted here because these terms will appear throughout, specifically the terms *adolescent, pornography*, and *Internet*.

Research on the impact of SEIM on youth has spanned a wide range of ages; however, there are some commonalities in the use of the term adolescent. Studies of adolescents and SEIM have examined the impact on children as young as 10 (Ybarra & Mitchell, 2005) and as old as 22 (Braun-Courville & Rojas, 2009). However, the majority of the research has focused the definition of adolescent to individuals between 13 and 18 years of age (e.g., Hunter, Figueredo, & Malamuth, 2010; Mesch, 2009; Peter & Valkenburg, 2006a, 2006b, 2008a, 2008b). While the information provided throughout this text may examine ages from childhood to adolescence, we will attempt to focus most of our attention on this 13- to 17-year-old population.

The other critical term that will be used throughout is pornography, sometimes referred to as *sexually explicit material*. If one looks at the term, both in scientific inquiry and in common vernacular, it is clear that defining pornography is a difficult and highly subjective process. The challenge in defining these terms was famously described by the U.S. Supreme Court Associate Justice Potter Stewart. In his concurring opinion in *Jacobellis v. Ohio* (1964), Justice Stewart wrote, "I shall not today attempt further to define the kinds of material I understand to be embraced within that shorthand description; and perhaps I could never succeed in intelligibly doing so. But I know it when I see it" ("Concurring Opinion of Mr. Justice Stewart," para. 1).

There are various descriptions of the term pornography throughout the literature. Peter and Valkenburg (2009) defined sexually explicit material as content "that depicts sexual activities in unconcealed ways, often with close-ups with (aroused) genitals and of oral, anal, or vaginal penetration" (p. 408). Tsitsika et al. (2009) defined pornographic Internet sites as "Internet sites portraying sexual behaviors and practices" (p. 546). Braun-Courville and Rojas (2009) defined sexually explicit websites as those that "describe people having sex, show clear pictures of nudity or people having sex, or show a movie or audio that describes people having sex" (p. 157).

For the purpose of this review, we will use the definition provided in the 1986 U.S. Attorney General Commission on Pornography. In that document, pornography was defined as any material that "is predominately sexually explicit and intended primarily for the purpose of sexual arousal" (McManus, 1986, p. 8).

Finally, we will attempt to define the Internet; rereading that sentence may cause some significant dissonance on the part of the reader, as it did on the part of the authors. In the not so distant past, the Internet was accessed through a desktop computer with an Internet Service Provider (ISP). It often involved the use of a telephone line and a dial-up modem. Speeds were slow and content was lacking by today's standards. While pornography was available, it was far less ubiquitous, and there was far less access. Downloading images via the Internet was a laborious process, one that may have been considered too difficult in comparison to other pornographic media, such as videos and magazines.

More recently, tablet computers, smartphones, video-game consoles, smart televisions, and other electronic devices have made the Internet available anytime, from anywhere. We can access the Internet using wireless technology in restaurants, shopping malls, and coffee shops. We do not need a dedicated connection to access the Internet; we can use cellular data available as we sit in a doctor's office or while watching a sporting event with 60,000 other fans. This unfettered access is noteworthy among adolescents. For example, a recent study found that one in three teenagers sends more than 100 text messages a day and 15% send more than 200 a day, or 6,000 a month (Lenhart et al., 2010. One study found that up to 60% of adolescents have sent or received a suggestive image to others (Peter & Valkenburg, 2016).

Because it is constantly changing, defining the Internet can be a Herculean task. While academic works rarely cite dictionary definitions, we feel it is appropriate in this case, given the succinct and clear definition provided by *Merriam-Webster*. According to Merriam-Webster (2019), the Internet is "an electronic communications network that connects computer networks and organizational computer facilities around the world" (para. 1).

Learning Activity 1.2 invites readers to consider how they access online material and to reflect on the ubiquitous nature of the Internet.

Learning Activity 1.2

How and when do you get online?

The Internet has become part of everyday life in ways we may not even consider. We invite you to reflect on the following question: how often do you access the Internet in a single day? Perhaps you keep a log throughout one day, from the time you wake until the time you sleep. Consider these questions:

- How did you access the Internet? (desktop computer, laptop computer, smartphone, tablet, gaming device, etc.)
- When did you access the Internet?
- For what purpose did you go online? (reading news, watching movies, checking sports scores, connecting with others via social media)
- How long were you online on each occasion?

As you begin to log these data, consider times you might be online and not thinking about it. For example, many of us will stream music in our vehicles or on mass transit while we commute. We can only do so by accessing the Internet. You might consider making note of those instances where you do not immediately realize you're online.

Prevalence of adolescents' use of SEIM

Studies examining adolescents' use consumption of SEIM have focused on three different areas: (1) unintentional use of SEIM, (2) intentional use, and (3) any use (i.e., both accidental and intended consumption of SEIM). Unintentional consumption of SEIM has been explored as both unwanted (e.g., Mitchell et al., 2003; Wolak, 2007) or accidental (e.g., Flood, 2007; Tsaliki, 2011). This type of consumption may occur when someone opens an email message, clicks on a website link, or searches for terms that may have unintended sexual meanings (e.g., searching for "Dick's Sporting Goods," a national chain of popular U.S.-based sporting goods stores). Prevalence rates for unintended consumption of SEIM ranged from 19% for 10- to 12-year-olds in the United States (Mitchell et al., 2003) to 84% for Australian boys aged 16–17 (Flood, 2007). In the United States, it is believed that prevalence rates of accidental or other unintentional SEIM use have dropped in recent years (Jones, Mitchell, & Finkelhor, 2012). More recent studies have found that 68% of U.S. teens had unintentionally viewed SEIM (Hardy, Steelman, Coyne, & Ridge, 2013).

When considering intentional use of SEIM, studies have explored situations where the consumption of SEIM was deliberate, often using specific, intentional terms in Internet searches (Peter & Valkenburg, 2016). Findings in the literature about the prevalence of intentional consumption have varied significantly. Ybarra and Mitchell (2005) found that 7% of 10- to 17-year-olds in the United States had intentionally consumed SEIM, while Chen, Leung, Chen, and Yang (2013) found that 59% of Taiwanese high schoolers had intentionally viewed SEIM. Similar divergent rates of prevalence were discovered when not accounting for intentionality. Rates of adolescent SEIM consumption worldwide suggest that nearly every adolescent has consumed SEIM, with some variance depending on the study, gender of the participants, country where the participants lived, and other factors (Peter & Valkenburg, 2016).

There are a number of limitations in the studies that have examined prevalence rates of adolescent SEIM consumption. First, most studies use self-report as a means of measuring prevalence; using this method, the adolescents who participate in these studies must be honest in their responses in order for researchers to collect accurate data. It can certainly be assumed that some young people may under-report their SEIM use out of embarrassment, moral judgments, legal concerns, and so forth. Additionally, many of the most recent studies are still dated, as there has not been much recent research on SEIM prevalence. Also, there are culture matters; some studies have been conducted in countries with more liberal attitudes about sex and SEIM, while other cultures may vary. Finally, many of these studies ask participants about one-time consumption of SEIM; these methods may not accurately reflect how SEIM use changes over time.

Regardless, the data certainly support the notion that adolescents consume SEIM. We know that adolescents have easy, ready access to the Internet, and the research suggests that they use this access, in part, to consume SEIM. The specific rates may be in question, but the notion that adolescents consume SEIM is not.

An overview of the text

The purpose of this text is to provide the reader with an overview of the most important issues related to young people and their consumption of Internet pornography. While the text is directed toward those in helping professions (e.g., counselors, psychologists, social workers, medical professionals, educators), we have tried to avoid a focus on any one specific profession where possible. Both authors identify as professional counselors in the United States; as a result, where a single profession is noted, for example in our review of ethics, we have provided examples from the counseling profession. However, there may be nuanced differences for other helping professions. We encourage the reader to consider how the information provided throughout can be applied to their own professions.

In Chapter 2, we take a step back from discussion of pornography specifically and examine the generational and cultural differences in how we use and perceive the Internet and how these differences can impact our relationships with young people. We examine the helping relationship specifically and explore the concepts of digital natives and digital immigrants through a cultural lens. The three chapters that follow explore the academic research that discusses relationships between the consumption of SEIM by young people and potential negative outcomes.

In Chapter 3, we examine the relationships between youth consumption of SEIM and the development of attitudes, values, and beliefs. Much of the research in this area is focused on gender-stereotypical attitudes, beliefs about sexuality and sexual behavior, and values related to intimate relationships. In Chapter 4, we explore the relationships found in the research between consumption of SEIM and adolescent behaviors. This research has typically focused on behaviors related to high-risk sexual behavior, aggression, violence, and casual sex. In Chapter 5, we review the literature related to adolescent SEIM consumption and the development of self-image. Self-image includes topics such as how one views one's own physical self, perceptions of one's attractiveness to others, and overall self-esteem. While these four chapters are heavily focused on the research literature, we make every effort to tie the theory to the practice of helping adolescents develop and grow in positive ways.

Chapter 6 explores relationships between adolescent consumption of SEIM and larger cultural issues. Our focus in this chapter is to examine how issues such as age, gender, religion, political ideology, and sexual identity may relate to the use of SEIM by young people. In Chapter 7, we examine the legal and ethical issues that are critical to those who work in the helping professions as those issues relate to young people and Internet pornography. Chapter 8 explores a few current issues in this field. In this chapter, we take a deeper dive into the issues related to free speech and laws related to SEIM. We also explore technological advances that allow for the development of doctored images and videos that are undetectable to many people (known as *deepfakes*) and adolescent use of technology to send sexually explicit images and videos to one another (knows as *sexting*).

Finally, in Chapter 9, we attempt to bring these many pieces together and provide guidance for how helping professionals can use this information in the best ways possible. As we discussed previously, the purpose of this text is to provide readers with helpful information as they navigate the rough waters of working with adolescents. We know adolescents use the Internet, and we know they use it to access pornography. In the last chapter, we try to provide some context as to how we can help the members of this population as they navigate those same rough waters.

Conclusion

This chapter provided an introduction to the text that follows. The structure and scope of the book was discussed, as well as how different terminology will be used throughout. The goal was to provide readers with a framework that will be important as they progress through the remainder of the book. We explored the significant prevalence of the Internet in the lives of young people around the world, as well as how this population uses technology to access sexually explicit material online. The data are clear; the Internet is ubiquitous in our world, and even more so in the lives of young people. This chapter provides the background that frames the information that follows.

Summary

- The purpose of this book is to provide insights and information about Internet pornography to helpers (counselors, psychologists, medical professionals, social workers, teachers, etc.) who work with adolescents.
- Over the past three decades, pornography has become far more commonplace than at any other point in history. The Internet has played a significant role in this mainstreaming of pornography, providing unequaled access to encounter, consume, create, and distribute sexually explicit content.
- Adolescents are most often still grappling with tasks related to executive functioning and may have difficulty prioritizing, making good decisions, and mitigating potential risks.
- Research on the impact of SEIM on youth has spanned a wide range of ages; however, there are some commonalities in the use of the term adolescent. For the purposes of this text, most references to adolescents will include those between 13 and 18 years of age.
- Pornography was defined in 1986 by the U.S. attorney general as any material that "is predominately sexually explicit and intended primarily for the purpose of sexual arousal" (McManus, 1986, p. 8).
- More recently, tablet computers, smartphones, video-game consoles, smart televisions, and other electronic devices have made the Internet available anytime, from anywhere.
- The Internet is "an electronic communications network that connects computer networks and organizational computer facilities around the world" (Merriam-Webster, 2019, para. 1).
- Prevalence rates of adolescent consumption of SEIM vary across research studies based on a number of factors (e.g., gender, culture, methodology). However, the fact that the adolescents consume SEIM is not in question.

Additional resources

In print

McManus, M. (1986). *Final report of the Attorney General's Commission on Pornography*. Nashville, TN: Rutledge Hill Press.

Paul, P. (2005). *Pornified: How pornography is transforming our lives, our relationships, and our families*. New York: Times Books.

On the web

Lenhart, A., Ling, R., Campbell, S., & Purcell, K. (2010). *Teens and mobile phones*. Washington, DC: Pew Research Center. Retrieved from http://pewinternet.org/~/media//Files/Reports/2010/PIP-Teens-and-Mobile-2010-with-topline.pdf

Roberts, D. F., Foehr, U. G., & Rideout, V. (2005). *Generation M: Media in the lives of 8–18 year olds*. Menlo Park, CA: The Henry J. Kaiser Family Foundation. Retrieved from www.kff.org/entmedia/upload/Generation-M-Media-in-the-Lives-of-8-18-Year-olds-Report.pdf

References

Barak, A., & Fisher, W. (2001). Toward an internet-driven, theoretically-based, innovative approach to sex education. *Journal of Sex Research*, *38*(4), 324–332. doi:10.1080/00224490109552103

Braun-Courville, D. K., & Rojas, M. (2009). Exposure to sexually explicit web sites and adolescent sexual attitudes and behaviors. *Journal of Adolescent Health*, *45*, 156–162. doi:10.1016/j.jadohealth.2008.12.004

Chen, A. S., Leung, M., Chen, C. H., & Yang, S. C. (2013). Exposure to Internet pornography among Taiwanese adolescents. *Social Behavior and Personality*, *41*, 157–164. doi:10.2224/sbp.2013.41.1.157

Cooper, A., Boies, S., Maheu, M., & Greenfield, D. (1999). Sexuality and the Internet: The next sexual revolution. In F. Muscarella & L. Szuchman (Eds.), *The psychological science of sexuality: A research-based approach* (pp. 519–545). New York: Wiley.

Coopersmith, J. (2006). Does your mother know what you *really* do? The changing image and nature of computer-based pornography. *History and Technology*, *22*(1), 1–25. doi:10.1080/07341510500508610

Delmonico, D. L., & Griffin, E. J. (2008). Cybersex and the E-Teen: What marriage and family therapists should know. *Journal of Marital and Family Therapy*, *34*(4), 431–444.

Flood, M. (2007). Exposure to pornography among youth in Australia. *Journal of Sociology*, *43*, 45–60. doi:10.1177/1440783307073934

Fu, K.-W., Chan, W. S. C., Wong, P. W. C., & Yip, P. S. F. (2010). Internet addiction: Prevalence, discriminant validity and correlates among adolescents in Hong Kong. *The British Journal of Psychiatry*, *196*, 486–492. doi:10.1192/bjp.bp.109.075002

Gillespie, A. A. (2008). Adolescents accessing indecent images of children. *Journal of Sexual Aggression*, *14*(2), 111–122. doi:10.1080/13552600802248122

Gómez, P., Rial, A., Braña, T., Golpe, S., & Varela, J. (2017). Screening of problematic internet use among Spanish adolescents: Prevalence and related variables. *Cyberpsychology, Behavior, and Social Networking*, *20*(4), 259–267. doi:10.1089/cyber.2016.0262

Häggström-Nordin, E., Sandberg, J., Hanson, U., & Tydén, T. (2006). "It's everywhere!" Young Swedish people's thoughts and reflections about pornography. *Scandinavian Journal of Caring Science*, *20*, 386–393. doi:10.1111/j.1471-6712.2006.00417.x

Hardy, S. A., Steelman, M. A., Coyne, S. M., & Ridge, R. D. (2013). Adolescent religiousness as a protective factor against pornography use. *Journal of Applied Developmental Psychology*, *34*, 131–139. doi:10.1016/j.appdev.2012.12.002

Hunter, J. A., Figueredo, A. J., & Malamuth, N. M. (2010). Developmental pathways into social and sexual deviance. *Journal of Family Violence*, *25*, 141–148. doi:10.1007/s10896-009-9277-9

Jacobellis v. Ohio, 368 U.S. 184 (1964).

Jones, L. M., Mitchell, K. L., & Finkelhor, D. (2012). Trends in youth Internet victimization: Findings from three youth Internet safety surveys. *Journal of Adolescent Health*, *50*, 179–186. doi:10.1016/j.jadolhealth.2011.09.015

Kawabe, K., Horiuchi, F., Ochi, M., Oka, Y., & Ueno, S. (2016). Internet addiction: Prevalence and relation with mental states in adolescents. *Psychiatry and Clinical Neurosciences*, *70*(9), 405–412. doi:10.1111/pcn.12402

Lam, L. T., Peng, Z., Mai, J.-C., & Jing, J. (2009). Factors associated with Internet addiction among adolescents. *CyberPsychology & Behavior*, *12*(5), 551–555. doi:10.1089=cpb.2009.0036

Lawsky, D. (2008). *American youth trail in Internet use: Survey*. Retrieved from reuters.com/article/us-internet-youth/american-youth-trail-in-internet-use-survey-idUSTRE4AN0MR20081124

Lenhart, A., Ling, R., Campbell, S., & Purcell, K. (2010). *Teens and mobile phones*. Washington, DC: Pew Research Center. Retrieved from http://pewinternet.org/~/media//Files/Reports/2010/PIP-Teens-and-Mobile-2010-with-topline.pdf

Lenhart, A., Purcell, K., Smith, A., & Zickur, K. (2010). Social media & mobile Internet use among teens and young adults. *PewInternet: Pew Internet & American Life Project*. Retrieved from http://pewinternet.org/Reports/2010/Social-Media-and-Young-Adults.aspx

Lo, V.-H., & Wei, R. (2005). Exposure to Internet pornography and Taiwanese adolescents' sexual attitudes and behavior. *Journal of Broadcasting and Electronic Media, 49*, 221–237. doi:10.1207/s15506878jobem4902_5

Löfgren-Mårtenson, L., & Månsson, S. (2010). Lust, love, and life: A qualitative study of Swedish adolescents' perceptions and experiences with pornography. *Journal of Sex Research, 47*, 568–579. doi:10.1080/00224490903151374

McManus, M. (1986). *Final report of the Attorney General's Commission on Pornography*. Nashville, TN: Rutledge Hill Press.

McNair, B. (2002). *Striptease culture: Sex, media and the democratization of desire*. London: Routledge.

Merriam-Webster. (2019). *Definition of Internet*. Retrieved from www.merriam-webster.com/dictionary/Internet

Mesch, G. S. (2009). Social bonds and Internet pornographic exposure among adolescents. *Journal of Adolescence, 32*, 601–618. doi:10.1016/j.adolescence.2008.06.004

Mitchell, K. J., Finkelhor, D., & Wolak, J. (2003). The exposure of youth to unwanted sexual material on the Internet: A national survey of risk, impact, and prevention. *Youth and Society, 34*, 330–358. doi:10.1177/0044118X02250123

Mitchell, K. J., Wolak, J., & Finkelhor, D. (2007). Trends in youth reports of sexual solicitations, harassment and unwanted exposure to pornography on the Internet. *Journal of Adolescent Health, 40*, 116–126. doi:10.1016/j.jadohealth.2006.05.021

Paul, P. (2005). *Pornified: How pornography is transforming our lives, our relationships, and our families*. New York: Times Books.

Peter, J., & Valkenburg, P. M. (2006a). Adolescents' exposure to sexually explicit online material and recreational attitudes toward sex. *Communication Research, 56*, 639–660. doi:10.1111/j.1460-2466.2006.00313.x

Peter, J., & Valkenburg, P. M. (2006b). Adolescents' exposure to sexually explicit material on the internet. *Journal of Communication, 33*, 178–204. doi:10.1177/0093650205285369

Peter, J., & Valkenburg, P. M. (2007). Adolescents' exposure to a sexualized media environment and notions of women as sex objects. *Sex Roles, 56*, 381–395. doi:10.1007/s11199-006-9176-y

Peter, J., & Valkenburg, P. M. (2008a). Adolescents' exposure to sexually explicit Internet material and sexual preoccupancy: A three-wave panel study. *Media Psychology, 11*, 207–234. doi:10.1080/15213260801994238

Peter, J., & Valkenburg, P. M. (2008b). Adolescents' exposure to sexually explicit Internet material, sexual uncertainty, and attitudes toward uncommitted sexual exploration: Is there a link? *Communication Research, 35*, 579–601. doi:10.1177/0093650208321754

Peter, J., & Valkenburg, P. M. (2009). Adolescents' exposure to sexually explicit Internet material and notions of women as sex objects: Assessing causality and underlying processes. *Journal of Communication, 59*, 407–433. doi:10.1111/j.1460-2466.2009.01422.x

Peter, J., & Valkenburg, P. (2016). Adolescents and pornography: A review of 20 years of research. *The Journal of Sex Research, 53*(4–5), 509–531. doi:10.1080/00224499.2016.1143441

Rimington, D., & Gast, J. (2007). Cybersex use and abuse: Implications for health education. *American Journal of Health Education, 38*(1), 34–40. doi:10.1080/19325037.2007.10598940

Roberts, D. F., Foehr, U. G., & Rideout, V. (2005). *Generation M: Media in the lives of 8–18 year olds*. Menlo Park, CA: The Henry J. Kaiser Family Foundation. Retrieved from www.kff.org/entmedia/upload/Generation-M-Media-in-the-Lives-of-8-18-Year-olds-Report.pdf

Rumpf, H. J., Vermulst, A. A., Bischof, A., Kastirke, N., Gürtler, D., Bischof, G., . . . Meyer, C. (2014). Occurrence of internet addiction in a general population sample: A latent class analysis. *European Addiction Research, 20*(4), 8. doi:10.1159/000354321

Sabina, C., Wolak, J., & Finkelhor, D. (2008). The nature and dynamics of Internet pornography exposure for youth. *CyberPsychology & Behavior, 11*(6), 691–693. doi:10.1089/cpb.2007.0179

Sussman, S. (2007). Sexual addiction among teens: A review. *Sexual Addiction & Compulsivity, 14*, 257–278. doi:10.1080/10720160701480758

Tsaliki, L. (2011). Playing with porn: Greek children's explorations in pornography. *Sex Education, 11*, 293–302. doi:10.1080/14681811.2011.590087

Tsitsika, A., Critselis, E., Kormas, D., Konstantoulaki, E., Constantopoulos, A., & Kafetzis, D. (2009). Adolescent pornographic Internet site use: A multivariate regression analysis of the predictive factors of use and psychosocial implications. *CyberPsychology and Behavior, 12*, 545–550. doi:10.1089=cpb.2008.0346

van den Eijnden, R. J. J. M., Spijkerman, R., Vermulst, A. A., van Rooij, T. J., & Engels, R. C. M. E. (2010). Compulsive Internet use among adolescents: Bidirectional parent-child relationships. *Journal of Abnormal Child Psychology, 38*, 77–89. doi:10.1007/s10802-009-9347-8

Villella, C., Martinotti, G., Di Nicola, M., Cassano, M., La Torre, G., Gliubizzi, M. D., . . . Conte, G. (2011). Behavioural addictions in adolescents and young adults: Results from a prevalence study. *Journal of Gambling Studies, 27*(2), 203–214. doi:10.1007/s10899-010-9206-0

Wolak, J., Mitchell, K., & Finkelhor, D. (2007). Unwanted and wanted exposure to online pornography in a national sample of youth Internet users. *Pediatrics, 119*, 247–257. doi:10.1542/peds.2006-1891

Ybarra, M. L., & Mitchell, K. J. (2005). Exposure to Internet pornography among children and adolescents: A national survey. *CyberPsychology and Behavior, 8*, 473–486. doi:10.1089/cpb.2005.8.473

Yen, C.-F., Ko, C.-H., Yen, J.-Y., Chang, Y.-P., & Cheng, C.-P. (2009). Multi-dimensional discriminative factors for Internet addiction among adolescents regarding gender and age. *Psychiatry and Clinical Neurosciences, 63*(3), 357–364. doi:10.1111/j.1440-1819.2009.01969.x

2 The digital divide

Strangers in a strange land

I just finished a therapy session with a new client named Rose. She's 14 years old and sits down across from me in the therapy room with her phone in her hand. As I start asking her some basic intake questions, she answers them but never looks up from her phone. It's like she's not even paying attention to me, and the whole point of her being here is because she's been sending inappropriate texts to boys in school. It's just rude, especially a girl of her age being so disrespectful to an adult.

Generational differences are always stark because, by definition, generations are different from one another based on important criteria. The vignette provides an example of the kind of generational differences that can be present in a counseling relationship. Parry and Urwin (2011) define a generation as "a set of historical events and related phenomena that creates a distinct generational gap" (p. 84). Generations are defined by social proximity to shared experiences. Research suggests that technology has been a defining feature of the most recent generations – a construct that will be discussed throughout the remainder of this text.

Understanding the differences in how generations appreciate and interact with technology can be crucial to quality helping relationships. As a result, in this chapter, we have chosen to focus on generational differences in the use of, and understanding of, technology, as well as how those differences impact the helping relationship. This chapter examines technology from a wider view and its place among adolescents, with less focus on pornography and SEIM specifically. The purpose of this chapter is to help the reader better understand how technology and culture intersect and how generational differences can impact the helping relationship.

After reading this chapter you should be able to

1 Define the different living generations;
2 Understand what makes younger generations unique, especially in relation to the use of technology;
3 Recognize the differences between digital natives and digital immigrants; and
4 Appreciate how younger generations perceive technology use, especially within the helping milieu.

Generations, defined

Any attempt to define a generation is unscientific, at best. The U.S. Census Bureau does not make such distinctions, with the exception of the definition of *Baby Boomers*. The Census Bureau defines this generation as being born between 1946 and 1964 (Colby & Ortman, 2014), which was the generation that followed the *Silent Generation*, born between 1922–1945 (Taylor & Keeter, 2010). Definitions beyond Baby Boomer become complicated and less distinct. Most researchers agree on a common term for the generation that followed the Baby Boomers, referred to as *Generation X*. The time frame that encompasses Generation X, however, is less clear, but is often defined as those who were born at the end of the Baby Boom generation through the early 1980s, most commonly 1981 or 1982 (Masnick, 2012).

The next generation has been called *Generation Y* by some but is more often referred to as the *Millennial* generation. Howe and Strauss (2000) defined Millennials in their seminal work, *Millennials Rising: The Next Generation*, as those born between 1982–2004. However, more recent definitions place the end of the Millennial generation around 1994 or 1995, with the generation that followed commonly referred to as *Generation Z*, the *iGeneration*, or the *9/11 Generation* (Turner, 2015). While terminology and specific date ranges may vary, it is widely understood that part of what makes a generation unique is that each has its own period of time, which is characterized by its own values, norms, and formative experiences.

As this text focuses on the Millennial generation and Generation Z, it is helpful to examine the specific values and norms that make these generations unique. Howe and Strauss (2000) and Reith (2005) describe the Millennial generation as more conventional than previous generations. Their relationships with parents and other authorities tend to be more positive than those of past generations, marked by greater degrees of trust. As the most loved and wanted generation in history (Dungy, 2011), Millennials have had more value placed on them, which has contributed to members of this generation having a sense of safety, as well as being special and having marked achievements (Twenge, 2010). This has led to greater degrees of overprotection by parents and society and lesser degrees of personal responsibility among Millennials.

Millennials take on adult roles later in life as a result of the excessive involvement of parents (Howe & Strauss, 2000). Millennials have highly structured schedules resulting from involvement in a multitude of activities (Reith, 2005) and tend to work from schedules and follow rules (Howe & Strauss, 2000; Lancaster & Stillman, 2002). This generation is perceived as dependent on others for problem solving, with a tendency to ignore problems in the hope that they will disappear (Much, Wagener, Breitkreutz, & Hellenbrand, 2014). And though this generation values structure and rules, their sense of being special may account for the perception that Millennial students think they will be exempt from following rules while expecting everyone else to follow them (Much et al., 2014).

Millennials have had greater exposure to technology, having been the center of home videos for years. This generation was the first to have widespread access to social media, chat rooms, and blogs. This has led to higher degrees of multitasking and a preference for team-oriented work (Howe & Strauss, 2000). Several researchers have found that members of this generation score higher on assessments of narcissism than did members of previous generations (Davenport, Bergman, Bergman, & Fearrington, 2014; Mehdizadeh, 2010; Twenge, 2010).

For comparison, members of Generation Z are more diverse than previous generations, with biracial and multiracial children representing the fastest growing segment of the U.S. population (American Academy of Adolescent Psychiatry, 2011). Sexuality is a more commonly accepted topic of discussion among Generation Z, and there are more Generation Z members of the lesbian, gay, bisexual, transgender, queer or questioning (LGBTQ) community than among previous generations (Turner, 2015). Generation Z is a more urban generation, with greater exposure to diversity than those who came before them.

Generation Z has been raised during a period where the middle class is shrinking and the income gap is growing (Turner, 2015). This generation has also been raised during a time of war (Tulgan, 2012); the oldest members of Generation Z were young children during the terrorist attacks of September 11, 2001, and the subsequent wars in Afghanistan and Iraq. As children raised in war and with economic uncertainty, Generation Z may feel less safe than previous generations. Most importantly for our analysis, Generation Z is the most comfortable and proficient generation in terms of the use of technology (Palley, 2012).

Digital immigrants and digital natives

Of importance to the current discussion is the influence of technology in the lives of later generations. There is much attention in the literature to how technology plays a prominent role in the lives of Millennials and Generation Z (Hazlett, 2008; Prensky, 2001; Reith, 2005). When examining Millennials in their adolescence, Lenhart, Purcell, Smith, and Zickuhr (2010) found that 93% of this population reported using the Internet regularly, and 73% of teens reported using social networking sites on a regular basis. When examining the same population, Lenhart (2012) found that 75% of adolescents in the United States report texting as their primary form of communication.

When examining Generation Z, Palley (2012) argues that this group is the first to be raised in a truly mobile era. Rideout, Foehr, and Roberts (2010) found that Generation Z youth spend more time engaged with media than any other activity besides sleeping. Between 2004 and 2009, the amount of time adolescents spent consuming media increased 67 minutes (Rideout et al., 2010). This is attributed in large part to the ubiquitous nature of the smartphone, which is now available to more children and adolescents than ever before, regardless of social class or socioeconomic status (Rideout et al., 2010).

As these trends began at the turn of the 21st century, Prensky (2001) made a significant distinction in the use of technology across generations. Specifically, he suggested that technology could be considered a cultural construct and suggested the terms *digital native* and *digital immigrant* to refer to how one consumes and considers technology in day-to-day life. The notion of the digital native resulted from Prensky's (2001) observation that the dissimilarities between these newer generations and those that preceded it are fundamentally different. He argues that members of newer generations "have not just changed *incrementally* from those of the past, nor simply changed their slang, clothes, body adornments, or styles . . . a really big *discontinuity* has taken place" (Prensky, 2001, p. 1). He points out that Millennials, and later Generation Z, were the first to be surrounded by new technologies from video games to cell phones, tablets, and other digital devices. These generations do not know a world without computers, email, the Internet, cell phones, and instant responses to questions.

Prensky's (2001) conclusion is that these fundamental generational differences have resulted in equally fundamental differences in the ways we think and process information. His use of the term digital native is intentional, because he examines this generational difference from a cultural perspective. Millennials are native to this culture; they speak a particular language, understand their environments through a different worldview, think in different ways, attack problems differently, communicate differently, and generally live differently than those from previous generations.

Prensky (2001) recognizes that for those individuals who are not digital natives – that is, those who were not born into this technological culture, there must be a different way of thinking about these previous generations. For previous generations, Prensky (2001) uses the term digital immigrant. The distinction is critical to his argument:

> As Digital Immigrants learn – like all immigrants, some better than others – to adapt to their environment, they always retain, to some degree, their "accent," that is, their foot in the past. The "digital immigrant accent" can be seen in such things as turning to the Internet second rather than first, or in reading the manual for a program rather than assuming the program will teach us how to use it. Today's older folk were "socialized" differently from their kids, and are now in the process of learning a new language. And a language learned later in life, scientists tell us, goes into a different part of the brain.
>
> (Prensky, 2001, p. 2)

Prensky (2001) identifies a variety of different examples of the accents found among digital immigrants. These include printing out your email or having someone else print it for you, printing documents for editing rather than editing via computer, asking people to view an interesting website on your device rather than sending a link, or even calling someone to ask if they received your email. The point Prensky (2001) is making with this distinction is that regardless of how much immigrants want to be natives, or how hard they may work at it, their accents will always give them away. As such, they can never truly be a part of that other culture because it is not native to them, and they will always carry their own native accent, which distinguishes them as separate from the digital native culture.

Prensky (2001) defined digital natives as those born after 1980, aligning closely with Howe and Strauss's (2000) definition of the Millennial. However, others have further delineated the digital native into various subgenerations. Helsper and Eynon (2010) referred to those born between 1980–1990 as first-generation digital natives. They further defined those born after 1990 as second-generation digital natives. Wang, Hsu, Campbell, Coster, and Longhurst (2014) identified a third generation of digital natives as those born after 2000. While the distinctions may seem arbitrary, they are based on significant distinctions between these subgenerations of digital natives and closely follow the loose definitions of Millennials and Generation Z.

The first-generation digital native was the first to interact regularly with a personal computer and perhaps the very beginning of what we now know as the Internet; however, neither was well developed nor even closely resembles what we see today. The second-generation digital native used Google, email, chat rooms, instant messaging, and iPods, a significant difference from their predecessors. The most recent generation of digital natives has a multitude of technological tools at their disposal: smartphones, tablets, cloud computing, and social networking sites, just to name a few.

We can consider how this distinction, native versus immigrant, impacts adolescent consumption of pornography. As technology has become ubiquitous and a part of generational culture, so has pornography's role as a cultural phenomenon. Chapter 6 will explore the role pornography plays in various cultures, but it is important to note here that subsequent generations have become more comfortable with, and arguably dependent on, the Internet. As that has occurred, those later generations have also become more comfortable with, and expectant of, interacting with pornography online. Learning Activity 2.1 provides an opportunity for self-reflection around identifying as a digital native or digital immigrant.

Learning Activity 2.1

Are you a native or an immigrant?

You have now had an opportunity to consider Prensky's (2001) distinction between digital natives and digital immigrants. Consider the following questions:

1 Do you identify as a digital native or digital immigrant?
2 What data do you have to support your answer to the previous question?
3 Would other members of this group with which you identify agree with your conclusion?
4 What challenges do you face when communicating with members of the other group?

Popular culture and adolescents

Social learning theory (Bandura, 1971) suggests that children and adolescents learn about sexuality, in part, from observing how sexuality is depicted around them. This vicarious learning is especially true when we consider how sexual content is positively or negatively viewed through the lens of popular culture and various media. With the ubiquity of Internet availability and the increase of smartphone ownership, uncensored and unregulated media has become more accessible than ever before.

In past decades and prior to the introduction of Internet pornography, there was a clear distinction between pornographic material and popular culture. However, over time, the mainstreaming of sexuality has pushed media boundaries and presented itself in a much more overt fashion. As today's youth are part of a highly sexualized, less judgmental, and more open and accepting society, sexuality in popular culture has been marketed accordingly. For example, adolescents are the primary audience for music videos (Andsager & Roe, 2003). It is not uncommon to see increasing sexual references made for audiences of all ages in music, television, and news.

Media can disseminate messages about socially acceptable behavior and norms, especially in regard to sexuality. In turn, youth who are exposed to sexual content in the media may develop a deeper knowledge and more liberal attitudes toward sexuality. In such a highly sexualized culture, it is almost certain that youth will encounter some form of sexually explicit content through various types of media. Exposure to sexual media can happen either intentionally or unintentionally, but we can almost be certain that today's youth will be impacted in some way. For many helping professionals, the main consideration is how the impact of sexuality of various media (e.g., music, television, and news can impact an adolescent's developing sexual sense of self.

Music

Adolescence is a time when music will play an integral part of development through both socialization and expression; music can be a way to learn and experience culture. For example, many adolescents consider music videos to be relevant sources of information on current affairs (Stephens & Few, 2007) and occasionally emulate both the style and behaviors of the artists they watch (Ey, 2016). The distribution of music in popular culture can be disseminated through multiple broadcast forms, much more than any other type of media. Like everything in society, music has evolved over time and so has the culture for which it plays. Music that was once broadcasted over radio or video is more commonly being streamed or downloaded online by younger generations. Music icons do not need to be met backstage or followed on tour when adolescents can follow artists' fan pages on social media. Why go to a concert when you can watch it on YouTube?

Historically, music has been a medium to disseminate messages about sexuality (Levin & Kilbourne, 2008). As culture has increasingly become sexualized, the music industry has followed suit. Many adolescents familiar with contemporary music videos show a preference for those that contain sexual content (Ey, 2016). It is estimated that more than one-third of popular songs contain sexual content (Martino, Collins, Elliott, Strachman, Kanouse, & Berry, 2006; Primack, Gold, Schwartz, & Dalton, 2008) and more than half of music videos contain sexual images (Frisby & Aubrey, 2012).

While the intensity of sexually explicit conduct in music and video continues to test the boundaries of censorship, youth are frequently being exposed to a sexual script similar to what is being portrayed in pornography. Like most pornographic scripts, many music videos portray males in positions of power over females who are treated as sexual objects (Wright & Rubin, 2017); this aligns with many of the negative stereotypes around sexual attitudes found in SEIM (ter Bogt, Engels, Bogers, & Kloosterman, 2010). Many sexual scripts in music videos depict risky sexual behaviors, sexual violence against females, unrealistic representations of romantic relationships, and feed stereotypes that males are driven by sex and have sex at an earlier age and with multiple partners (Wright & Rubin, 2017).

Television

According to the U.S. Department of Labor (2018), roughly 80% of Americans watch television on any given day, including adolescents. Unlike the black and white television shows that were once watched on the one and only household television that sat mostly quiet in a family room, television shows can now be streamed live over the Internet and to mobile devices, anytime and anywhere. The exposure to televised media through means other than an actual television will only continue to increase with the development of online technology.

Television, regardless of the media in which it is received, has allowed sexual content to be broadcasted to youth of all ages, inadvertently redefining what many would consider normal age-appropriate programming for a child. For many youth, television and movies are thought to be some of the most informative sources of sexual education available (Bleakley, Hennessy, Fishbein, & Jordan, 2008), and what youth watch will have an influence on their daily attitudes, beliefs, and behaviors (Bleakley, Hennessy, & Fishbein, 2011).

For the most part, sexuality is portrayed on television as a positive experience. Very seldom are television actors portrayed in a negative light, and sexual behavior depicted on television rarely has any behavioral risks or consequences. For example, consider how often a physical relationship on television concludes with an unwanted pregnancy or a sexually transmitted infection. The answer is probably "rarely." It is possible that television portrayals of sexuality may lead youth to believe that sexual intercourse is a common recreational activity among peers (Ward & Friedman, 2006). However, it is rare to see television programs consider the emotional aspects of sexuality.

News

In 2018, pornography found its way to the forefront of American political coverage, receiving an unprecedented amount of attention online and in social media.

Adult film actress Stephanie Clifford, better known as Stormy Daniels, had alleged an extramarital affair in 2006 with now U.S. President Donald Trump. Clifford reported that she was given a cash payment as hush money in the days leading up to the 2016 presidential election, which later transpired into a dispute surrounding a nondisclosure agreement and a political scandal that would set the news cycle for months. Between the numerous appearances and interviews of Clifford and her attorney, the name "Porn Star Stormy Daniels" had become a household name in American politics.

In other news, adult film actress Carolyn Paparozzi, better known as Cherie DeVille, ended her 2020 presidential campaign (Nelson, 2019). Pornographic film star Jenna Massoli, better known as Jenna Jameson (2018), made headlines after she revealed on Instagram her 80-pound weight loss on the popular keto diet. These examples prove that one does not necessarily need to view pornography to be familiar with pornographic culture. As described earlier, the adult film industry is present in politics, current affairs, and popular weight-loss fads, among many other issues that make the news around the world.

The exposure of adolescents to various forms of sexually suggestive media has become normalized in today's popular culture. In the digital age, the consumption of music, television, and news have become increasingly accessed online and through social media. With the hypersexualization of musicians in popular culture, it can sometimes appear that pornography has overlaid popular culture with porn culture. For adolescents who are in a rapid period of personal development, exposure to content on television will almost certainly have an impact on how sexuality is portrayed and could potentially desensitize youth to SEIM. An adolescent does not need to consume SEIM to be familiar with the current affairs in pornography, as major news outlets are increasingly covering headlines from this industry. While adolescents may have access to sexual messages through a variety of media, including television, music, and news, the Internet remains the preferred way of seeking sexual information (Bleakley et al., 2011) and for the specific purpose of viewing pornography (Træen, Nilsen, & Stigum, 2006).

The digital native and the helping relationship

As we consider how best to provide helping services (e.g., counseling and psychological services, social work services), it is important to consider the relationships between generational differences, technology, and mental health. Hoffman (2013) examined these issues specific to the therapeutic relationship. She suggested that counselors who find themselves as digital immigrants working in the digitally native world of Millennials must take a culture-infused approach in order to be successful. Hoffman (2013) argued that culture is defined by aspects of one's life that are highly important, such as age, means of communication, and so forth. Using this definition, the significance of technology would help to define Millennials as a distinct culture, worthy of specific consideration.

Many adolescents believe that adults do not understand them; there is nothing new in this statement. However, with the explosion of technology over the past two decades, these feelings of misunderstanding can be exacerbated and lead to difficulty in connecting with younger generations. For example, Li (2010) found that only one in ten children or adolescents will report cyberbullying to adults for fear of the adult not understanding the concern. Adolescents may not want to discuss concerns with adults for fear that they will be misunderstood and therefore not taken seriously (Larsen & Ryberg, 2011). Consider the implications for counselors working with adolescents whose concerns relate to technology and sexuality; adolescents typically are not comfortable discussing sex and pornography with adults; the impact of technology may only serve to exacerbate this problem.

Hoffman (2013) argues, "Therapists should consider that when youth use social media, even in ways that adults perceive as deviant, they are engaging in behaviors that are normative for their culture" (p. 123). When providing interventions, it is critical that counselors consider their own cultural competence when working with clients. If we accept Hoffman's (2013) premise that technology's impact on adolescents is, in fact, a cultural phenomenon, then cultural competence becomes part of understanding this population's use of technology. The Multicultural Counseling and Social Justice Competencies (Ratts, Singh, Nassar-McMillan, Butler, & McCullough, 2016) propose that in order to provide culturally competent, effective counseling interventions, helpers must have knowledge of the cultural differences, such as those described previously. It is also critical to examine one's own attitudes and beliefs toward cultural differences. The learning activity that follows invites the reader to engage in this practice.

Learning Activity 2.2

Examining our own attitudes and beliefs about technology

This exercise is intended to challenge the reader to consider your knowledge, skills, and attitudes toward technology and pornography. Consider the following case example and then respond to the questions that follow.

Mr. Snyder is a clinical social worker who works with families that are in conflict. Recently, he began work with a family of four: father, mother, and two teenage daughters. The daughters have been in conflict with their parents since discovering that their parents have been viewing Internet pornography using the family's smart television. The teenage daughters describe themselves as "mortified" at the idea that their parents are using the family television to view what they describe as "perverse" videos online. The parents, while embarrassed, have been trying to explain to their children that such behavior is a healthy element of a sexual relationship between consenting adults. The teenage daughters have challenged their parents' perspective of "healthy," explaining that they believe many females in the pornography industry are victims of the objectification of females and a misogynistic culture.

Consider this case and the following questions:

1. How much do you know about the information presented in this case? Obviously, there is a difference of opinion; do you have any factual knowledge about either point of view?
2. What is your own attitude toward pornography, especially in terms of the arguments being made by the different parties in this case illustration?
3. How might your attitudes impact your work with this family? Should you consider bracketing your own perspectives?
4. If so, how will you go about trying to do so? If not, are their potential consequences to not trying to do so?

The following is provided to assist the reader in engaging in the last two elements of culturally competent counseling, developing skills and putting these pieces into action (Ratts et al., 2016). Specifically, we provide information on the use of technology when counseling adolescent populations. If we accept the premise that younger generations are the most technologically connected and are, therefore, digital natives, then how do adolescents interact with technology in relation to mental health?

The literature has swelled in recent years, with specific attention to issues such as problematic Internet use (Mitchell, Becker-Blease, & Finkelhor, 2005), Internet pornography (Owens, Behun, Manning, & Reid, 2012), psychological well-being (Kim, LaRose, & Peng, 2009), and personality issues (Amichai-Hamburger & Vinitzky, 2010). For example, Mitchell et al. (2005) surveyed over 1,500 mental health practitioners who worked with at least one client with an Internet-related concern. Their findings indicated 11 categories of problematic Internet use among both children and adults, including such issues as overuse, infidelity, sexual exploitation, gambling, fraud, and harassment. While SEIM was not a specific focus of this study, many of the areas of focus do intersect with the consumption of SEIM.

Kim et al. (2009) conducted a study of individuals who identified as lonely and lacking social skills. They found that these factors led to excessive and problematic use of the Internet. Specifically, this study found that individuals who identified as lonely had negative life outcomes as a result of Internet use, such as challenges related to work, school, and interpersonal relationships. Furthermore, their problematic Internet use led to a cycle of social isolation, leading to additional loneliness. As we consider the implications of this study on adolescent sexual development, it is easy to see how the findings related to loneliness might translate to SEIM and sexual development among adolescents.

Research findings in this area are not consistently negative, however. Boniel-Nissim and Barak (2013) examined the therapeutic value of using the Internet to journal about emotional challenges through the use of web logs, commonly referred to as blogs. The study examined six groups of 26–28 participants who were assessed as having social-emotional difficulties. Four of these groups blogged about their experiences; one group wrote a personal diary using a computer; the sixth group served as a control group that did not engage in either activity. The data suggested that those adolescents who maintained an online blog showed significant improvement on all of the assessed scales of social-emotional difficulty, self-esteem, social activity, and textual analyses of the blog posts. These findings could be important for therapists looking for creative outlets for adolescents who turn to technology as a primary outlet for emotional struggles.

Kennedy's (2014) investigation of TechnoWellness, "a mode of interacting with technology that maximizes its potential to enhance health and well-being and contribute to an optimal life" (p. 114), examined both the benefits and challenges of technology related to wellness and counseling. Kennedy (2014) developed an instrument to assess TechnoWellness: the TechnoWellness Inventory (TWI). TWI scores can inform practitioners about client wellness with respect to technology along the following domains: social self, creative self, coping self, essential self, and physical self. Kennedy (2015) identified five TechnoWellness factors assessed by the TWI: using technology for leisure, using technology for vocational purposes, technostress (e.g., stress over lack of technology skills, work bleeding into leisure space, feeling out of control or unmotivated by technology), using technology for physical health (e.g., using apps to monitor exercise, diet, and weight), and excess use of technology.

Kennedy (2014) proposed that assessment of client interactions with technology is the first step "to help someone make the best use of technology to achieve optimal health and well-being" (p. 122). Kennedy (2014, 2015) outlined several questions that can be used to assess the positive and negative effects of technology along the five wellness domains, thus informing counselor interventions aimed toward clients interacting with technology to foster wellness while raising client awareness of the role of technology in their presenting issues.

Other studies have examined how technology can be used as an adjunct to traditional therapeutic treatments. Youn et al. (2013) examined the use of Facebook as a screening tool for major depressive disorder (MDD). Specifically, college students at five universities were targeted for completion of an MDD assessment instrument, and resources for counseling were provided to those who indicated symptoms of MDD. Use of social media sites could be an opportunity for screening and early intervention with adolescents who may have concerns around sexuality and pornography consumption.

Clough and Casey (2011) examined the technological adjuncts available to augment face-to-face therapy. Specifically, they found that use of mobile phones, personal digital assistants, biofeedback, and virtual reality can enhance the practice of traditional face-to-face counseling. Riva, Baños, Botella, Wiederhold, and Gaggioli (2012) examined the use of technology in promoting positive psychology concepts, a cornerstone of the counseling profession. Using the term *positive technology*, these authors suggested that technology can provide the opportunity for individuals to improve affect, engagement, actualization, and connectedness.

Newman, Szkodny, Llera, and Przeworski (2011) examined the use of technology-assisted, self-help interventions in the treatment of anxiety and depression through a review of the literature on these issues. They found that self-help and self-administered technology-based interventions can be effective for motivated clients diagnosed with anxiety disorders. They also found that these minimal-contact interventions were effective in maintaining treatment compliance and reducing attrition in this clientele. Additionally, for clients who indicated symptoms of depression but did not meet the threshold for a diagnosed mood disorder, computer-based cognitive and behavioral interventions proved effective. However, for those who met the criteria for depression, therapist-assisted treatments proved the most effective.

Conclusion

Clearly, generational differences impact how we understand and interact with technology. Prensky's (2001) definitions of digital natives and digital immigrants provide important distinctions between generations and how each exists within the digital world that is simply unavoidable. If we consider the helping relationship from a cultural lens, as Hoffman (2013) suggests, then we can consider both how technology may impact different generational understandings of SEIM and ways we might consider treating adolescents who present with issues of depression, anxiety, or other concerns related to the consumption of SEIM. In short, if technology presents a challenge in working with adolescent populations, it may also offer some solutions, provided we are willing to consider our own perceptions of technology as compared to that of other generations'.

Summary

- A generation is defined as "a set of historical events and related phenomena that creates a distinct generational gap" (Parry & Urwin, 2011, p. 84).
- Millennials were born between 1982 and 1994 or 1995, with the generation that followed commonly referred to as *Generation Z*, the *iGeneration*, or the *9/11 Generation*.
- The Millennial generation is marked by positive relationships with parents, a sense of safety, decreased personal responsibility, a later ascension into adulthood, a value on rules, and dependence on others. Millennials were the first generation to be raised in the digital age.
- Generation Z is marked by greater diversity, less economic and personal safety, and the greatest comfort with technology.
- According to Prensky (2001), technology is a cultural construct; digital natives speak a particular language, understand their environments through a different worldview, think in different ways, attack problems differently, communicate differently, and generally live differently than those from previous generations.
- If technology is viewed through a cultural lens, what might be considered problematic or deviant to one culture might be considered normative to another.

- While adolescents may have access to sexual messages through a variety of media, including television, music, and news, the Internet remains the preferred way of seeking sexual information and for the specific purpose of viewing pornography.
- Technology has significant implications for helping processes. Technology has been found to correlate with some negative outcomes, such as loneliness and a lack of social skills. Technology may also have positive elements, such as its use in the helping process.

Additional resources

In print

Hoffman, A. (2013). Bridging the digital divide: Using culture-infused counseling to enhance therapeutic work with digital youth. *Journal of Infant, Child, and Adolescent Psychotherapy, 12*, 118–133.

Howe, N., & Strauss, W. (2000). *Millennials rising: The next great generation*. New York: Vintage Books.

Lancaster, L. C., & Stillman, D. (2002). *When generations collide: Who they are: Why the clash: How to solve the generational puzzle at work*. New York: Harper.

On the web

Colby, S. L., & Ortman, J. M. (2014). The baby boom cohort in the United States: 2012 to 2060: Population estimates and projections. *United States Census Bureau*. Retrieved from www.census.gov

Prensky, M. (2001). Digital natives, digital immigrants. *On the Horizon, 9*(6). Retrieved from www.marcprensky.com/writing/Prensky%20%20Digital%20Natives,%20Digital%20Immigrants%20-%20Part1.pdf

Rideout, V. J., Foehr, U. G., & Roberts, D. F. (2010, January). *Generation M2: Media in the lives of 8–18 year olds*. Menlo Park, CA: The Henry J. Kaiser Family Foundation. Retrieved from http://kaiserfamilyfoundation.files.wordpress.com/2013/01/8010.pdf

References

American Academy of Child and Adolescent Psychiatry. (2011). *Facts for families: Multiracial children*. Retrieved from www.aacap.org/App_Themes/AACAP/docs/facts_for_families/71_multiracial_children.pdf

Amichai-Hamburger, Y., & Vinitzky, G. (2010). Social network use and personality. *Computer in Human Behavior, 26*, 1289–1295. doi:10.1016/j.chb.2010.03.018

Andsager, J., & Roe, K. (2003). "What's your definition of dirty, baby?": Sex in music video. *Sexuality & Culture: An Interdisciplinary Quarterly, 7*(3), 79–97. https://doi.org/10.1007/s12119-003-1004-8

Bandura, A. (1971). *Social learning theory*. New York: General Learning Press.

Bleakley, A., Hennessy, M., & Fishbein, M. (2011). A model of adolescents' seeking of sexual content in their media choices. *Journal of Sex Research, 48*(4), 309–315. doi:10.1080/00224499.2010.497985

Bleakley, A., Hennessy, M., Fishbein, M., & Jordan, A. (2008). It works both ways: The relationship between exposure to sexual content in the media and adolescent sexual behavior. *Media Psychology, 11*, 443–461. doi:10.1080/15213260802491986

Boniel-Nissim, M., & Barak, A. (2013). The therapeutic value of adolescents' blogging about social-emotional difficulties. *Psychological Services, 10*, 333–341. doi:10.1037/a0026664

Clough, B. A., & Casey, L. M. (2011). Technological adjuncts to enhance current psychotherapy practices: A review. *Clinical Psychology Review, 31*, 279–292. doi:10.1016/j.cpr.2010.12.008

Colby, S. L., & Ortman, J. M. (2014). The baby boom cohort in the United States: 2012 to 2060: Population estimates and projections. *United States Census Bureau*. Retrieved from www.census.gov

Davenport, S. W., Bergman, S. M., Bergman, J. S., & Fearrington, M. E. (2014). Twitter versus Facebook: Exploring the role of narcissism in the motives and usage of different social media platforms. *Computers in Human Behavior, 32*, 212–220.

Dungy, G. J. (2011). Chapter I: A national perspective: Testing our assumptions about generational cohorts. In F. Bonner, II, A. F. Marbley, & M. F. Howard-Hamilton (Eds.), *Diverse millennial students in college: Implications for faculty and student affairs*. Sterling, VA: Stylus Publishing.

Ey, L.-A. (2016). Sexualized music media and children's gender role and self-identity development: A four-phase study. *Sex Education, 16*(6), 634–648. doi:10.1080/14681811.2016.1162148

Frisby, C. M., & Aubrey, J. S. (2012). Race and genre in the use of sexual objectification in female artists' music videos. *Howard Journal of Communications, 23*(1), 66–87. doi:10.1080/10646175.2012.641880

Hazlett, B. (2008, June). *Social networking statistics & trends* [Slideshare]. Retrieved from www.slideshare.net/onehalfamazing/social-networking-statistics-and-trends-presentation

Helsper, E. J., & Eynon, R. (2010). Digital natives: Where is the evidence? *British Educational Research Journal, 36*, 503–520. doi:10.1080/01411920902989227

Hoffman, A. (2013). Bridging the digital divide: Using culture-infused counseling to enhance therapeutic work with digital youth. *Journal of Infant, Child, and Adolescent Psychotherapy, 12*, 118–133. doi:10.1080/15289168.2013.791195

Howe, N., & Strauss, W. (2000). *Millennials rising: The next great generation*. New York: Vintage Books.

Jameson, J. [@jennacantlose]. (2018, July 23). *Photograph of before and after*. Retrieved from www.instagram.com/p/Bllno4IAIFR/?utm_source=ig_embed

Kennedy, S. D. (2014). TechnoWellness: A new wellness construct in the 21st century. *Journal of Counselor Leadership and Advocacy, 1*, 113–127. doi:10.1080/2326716X.2014.902759

Kennedy, S. D. (2015, April 28). *Wellness series: TechnoWellness: Exploring the relationship between technology use and wellness* [Webinar]. Retrieved from www.csi-net.org/default.asp?page=Webinars_Recorded

Kim, J., LaRose, R., & Peng, W. (2009). Loneliness as the cause and effect of problematic Internet use: The relationship between Internet use and psychological well-being. *CyberPsychology & Behavior, 12*, 451–455. doi:10.1089/cpb.2008.0327

Larsen, M. C., & Ryberg, T. (2011). Youth and online social networking: From local experiences to public disclosures. In E. Dunkels, G. M. Franberg, & C. Hallgren (Eds.), *Youth culture and net culture: Online social practices* (pp. 17–40). Hershey, PA: Information Science Reference.

Lenhart, A. (2012). Teens, smartphones and texting. *Pew Internet and American Life Project*. Retrieved from http:www.pewinternet.org/Reports/2012/Teens-and-smartphones/Summary-of-Findings.aspx

Lenhart, A., Purcell, K., Smith, A., & Zickuhr, K. (2010). Social media and young adults. *Pew Internet and American Life Project*. Retrieved from http:www.pewinternet.org/Reports/2010/Social-Media-and-Young-Adults/Summary-of-Findings.aspx

Levin, D. E., & Kilbourne, J. (2008). *So sexy so soon: The new sexualized childhood and what parents can do to protect their kids*. New York: Ballantine Books.

Li, Q. (2010). Cyberbullying in high schools: A study of students' behaviors and beliefs about this new phenomenon. *Journal of Aggression, Maltreatment & Trauma, 19*(4), 372–392. doi:10.1080/10926771003788979

Martino, S. C., Collins, R. L., Elliott, M. N., Strachman, A., Kanouse, D. E., & Berry, S. H. (2006). Exposure to degrading versus nondegrading music lyrics and sexual behavior among youth. *Pediatrics, 118*(2), 430–441. doi:10.1542/peds.2006-0131

Masnick, G. (2012, November 28). Defining the generations. *Joint Center for Housing Studies of Harvard University*. Retrieved from http://housingperspectives.blogspot.com/2012/11/defining-generations.html

Mehdizadeh, S. (2010). Self-presentation 2.0: Narcissism and self-esteem on Facebook. *Cyberpsychology, Behavior, and Social Networking, 13*, 357–364. doi:10.1089/cyber.2009.0257

Mitchell, K. J., Becker-Blease, K. A., & Finkelhor, D. (2005). Inventory of problematic Internet experiences encountered in clinical practice. *Professional Psychology: Research and Practice, 36*, 498–509. doi:10.1037/0735-7028.36.5.498

Much, K., Wagener, A. M., Breitkreutz, H. L., & Hellenbrand, M. (2014). Working with the millennial generation: Challenges facing 21st-century students from the perspective of university staff. *Journal of College Counseling, 17*, 37–47. doi:10.1002/j.2161-1882.2014.00046.x

Nelson, S. (2019, January 31). It's off: Porn star running for president thrown in the towel. *Washington Examiner*. Retrieved from www.washingtonexaminer.com/news/whitehouse/its-off-porn-star-running-for-president-throws-in-the-towel

Newman, M. G., Szkodny, L. E., Llera, S. J., & Przeworski, A. (2011). A review of technology-assisted self-help and minimal contact therapies for anxiety and depression: Is human contact necessary for therapeutic efficacy? *Clinical Psychology Review, 31*, 89–103. doi:10.1016/j.cpr.2010.09.008

Owens, E. W., Behun, R. J., Manning, J. C., & Reid, R. C. (2012). The impact of Internet pornography on adolescents: A review of the literature. *Sexual Addiction and Compulsivity: The Journal of Treatment and Prevention, 19*, 99–122. doi:10.1080/10720162.2012.660431

Palley, W. (2012). *Gen Z: Digital in their DNA*. New York, NY: Thompson. Retrieved from www.jwtintelligence.com/wpcontent/uploads/2012/04/F_INTERNAL_Gen_Z_0418122.pdf

Parry, E., & Urwin, P. (2011). Generational differences in work values: A review of theory and evidence. *International Journal of Management Reviews, 13*(1), 79–96. doi:10.1111/j.1468-2370.2010.00285.x

Prensky, M. (2001). Digital natives, digital immigrants. *On the Horizon, 9*(6). Retrieved from www.marcprensky.com/writing/Prensky%20%20Digital%20Natives,%20Digital%20Immigrants%20-%20Part1.pdf

Primack, B., Gold, M., Schwartz, E., & Dalton, M. (2008). Degrading and non-degrading sex in popular music: A content analysis. *Public Health Reports, 123*, 593–600. doi:10.1177/003335490812300509

Ratts, M. J., Singh, A. A., Nassar-McMillan, S., Butler, S. K., McCullough, J. R. (2016). Multicultural and social justice counseling competencies: Guidelines for the counseling profession. *Journal of Multicultural Counseling and Development, 44*(1), 28–48. doi:10.1002/jmcd.12035

Reith, J. (2005). Understanding and appreciating the communication styles of the millennial generation. In *Compelling perspectives on counseling: Vistas* (pp. 321–324). Retrieved from www.counseling.org/knowledge-center/vistas/vistas-2005

Rideout, V. J., Foehr, U. G., & Roberts, D. F. (2010, January). *Generation M2: Media in the lives of 8–18 year olds*. Menlo Park, CA: The Henry J. Kaiser Family Foundation. Retrieved from http://kaiserfamilyfoundation.files.wordpress.com/2013/01/8010.pdf

Riva, G., Baños, R. M., Botella, C., Wiederhold, B. K., & Gaggioli, A. (2012). Positive technology: Using interactive technologies to promote positive functioning. *Cyberpsychology, Behavior, and Social Networking, 15*, 69–77. doi:10.1089/cyber.2011.0139

Stephens, D. P., & Few, A. L. (2007). Hip hop honey or video ho: African American preadolescents' understanding of female sexual scripts in hip hop culture. *Sexuality & Culture: An Interdisciplinary Quarterly, 11*(4), 48–69. doi:10.1007/s12119-007-9012-8

Taylor, P., & Keeter, S. (2010). *Millennials: A portrait of generation next*. Washington, DC: Pew Research Center. Retrieved from://www.pewsocialtrends.org

ter Bogt, T. F. M., Engels, R. C. M. E., Bogers, S., & Kloosterman, M. (2010). "Shake it baby, shake it": Media preferences, sexual attitudes and gender stereotypes among adolescents. *Sex Roles: A Journal of Research, 63*, 844–859. doi:10.1007/s11199-010-9815-1

Træen, B., Nilsen, T. S., & Stigum, H. (2006). Use of pornography in traditional media and on the Internet in Norway. *Journal of Sex Research, 43*(3), 245–254. doi:10.1080/00224490609552323

Tulgan, B. (2012, June 26). *High-maintenance Generation Z heads to work*. USA Today. Retrieved from http://usatoday30.usatoday.com/news/opinion/forum/story/2012-06-27/generation-z-work-millenials-social-media-graduates/55845098/1

Turner, A. (2015). Generation Z: Technology and social interest. *The Journal of Individual Psychology, 71*(2), 103–113. doi:10.1353/jip.2015.0021

Twenge, J. M. (2010). A review of empirical evidence on generational differences in work attitudes. *Journal of Business Psychology, 25*, 201–210. doi:10.1007/s10869-010-9165-6

United States Department of Labor, Bureau of Labor Statistics. (2018). *Television, capturing America's attention at prime time and beyond*. Retrieved from www.bls.gov/opub/btn/volume-7/televisioncapturing-americas-attention.htm

Wang, S., Hsu, H., Campbell, T., Coster, D. C., & Longhurst, M. (2014). An investigation of middle school science teachers and students use of technology inside and outside of classrooms: Considering whether digital natives are more technologically savvy than their teachers. *Education Technology Research and Development, 62*, 637–662. doi:10.1007/s11423-014-9355-4

Ward, M. L., & Friedman, K. (2006). Using TV as a guide: Associations between television viewing and adolescents' sexual attitudes and behavior. *Journal of Research on Adolescence, 16*, 133–156. doi:10.1111/j.1532-7795.2006.00125.x

Wright, C. L., & Rubin, M. (2017). "Get lucky"! Sexual content in music lyrics, videos and social media and sexual cognitions and risk among emerging adults in the USA and Australia. *Sex Education, 17*(1), 41–56. doi:10.1080/14681811.2016.1242402

Youn, S. J., Trinh, N.-H., Shyu, I., Change, T., Fava, M., Kvedar, J., & Yeung, A. (2013). Using online social media, Facebook, in screening for major depressive disorder among college students. *International Journal of Clinical Health Psychology, 13*, 74–80. doi:10.1016/S1697-2600(13)70010-3

3 Thoughts and values
Pornography and attitudes and beliefs

Cheryl is a 17-year-old female who is sitting in the therapy room discussing her fears related to becoming sexually active with her new boyfriend. "I've always believed that sex should be something special, something intimate. I know that guys don't always see it that way, and that's fine. But to me, I want it to matter. I'm not saying I'm going to wait until marriage, but it seems like people my age don't think like I do. My friends, guys and girls, all watch porn, and it's like it makes them think that sex is less important than it should be. But maybe they're right? Maybe it's not a big deal. My parents always raised me to think that it should be something I wait to do until I'm really in love, but no one else seems to care about that.

An area of research that has received significant attention is the relationship between young people's consumption of SEIM and their attitudes and beliefs about sex and relationships. Attitudes and beliefs are broad terms, difficult to define, but much of the research has examined how adolescents think about the opposite sex, their own bodies and sexuality, and their attitudes about engaging in sexual behavior. It should be noted that attitudes and beliefs are different from behaviors, which will be discussed in more detail in the next chapter. Certainly, they may be related; if teenagers have the belief that sexual activity is acceptable, then they may be more likely to engage in that activity. But attitudes and beliefs, in and of themselves, do not equate to behavior.

In this chapter, we examine the relationships between SEIM and the thoughts and feelings of adolescents about sex and sexuality. The vignette at the opening is intended to raise awareness of these issues. Adolescence is a time of development, physically, cognitively, and emotionally. Thoughts and feelings are in a constant state of flux during this time, and the messages young people receive can certainly help to shape those attitudes and beliefs. When one's personal belief system is challenged by those external messages and dissonance results, it is the role of helping professionals to guide adolescents through that internal conflict.

After reading this chapter, you should be able to

1 Appreciate the relationships found in the research between adolescent consumption of SEIM and attitudinal changes;
2 Understand the different types of attitudes and beliefs that relate to adolescent sexuality and how each is related to SEIM use; and

3   Develop intervention strategies to address unhealthy attitudes and beliefs in adolescents that may result from SEIM consumption.

The Centerfold Syndrome

In his book *Clinical Psychology*, Gary Brooks (1995) identifies a phenomenon he refers to as "the Centerfold Syndrome." Brooks (1995) suggests that heterosexual male sexuality is largely driven by media, and the effect that media has on men leads them to objectify females. The author goes on to posit that males are socialized through media to develop five specific sets of beliefs or attitudes. Wright (2012) provides five labels for these sets of beliefs: (1) voyeurism, (2) sexual reductionism, (3) masculinity validation, (4) trophyism, and (5) nonrelational sex.

The term *voyeurism*, in this context, refers to the belief that seeing others as sexual objects is natural and unavoidable (Brooks, 1995). To view others sexually (i.e., in pornography or other forms of media) is inevitable and a regular part of the male experience. *Sexual reductionism* refers to the attitude that females are to be evaluated on their sexual appeal and their physical appearance (Brooks, 1995). The theory suggests that through media consumption, males are socialized to value females as sexual objects, measured by their attractiveness. *Masculinity validation* suggests that males can validate their worth through females – specifically that one's sense of being male or masculine is validated through sexual conquest and the male's ability to please a female partner sexually. *Trophyism* refers to the belief that females can be used as trophies to gain social status (Brooks, 1995). The theory speculates that males can gain approval from other men, and perhaps females, by "acquiring" an attractive female partner or mate. Finally, *nonrelational sex* identifies a belief that through consuming sexualized media, males are more apt to believe that sexual behavior is recreational and nonrelational (Brooks, 1995). This theory suggests that males learn to depersonalize the sexual relationship and view it as merely fun.

While the Centerfold Syndrome has been widely cited and discussed throughout the literature, it has historically lacked empirical support to confirm its generalizability (Barbee, 1997, 1998). As a result, Wright and Tokunaga (2015) conducted a study with college-aged, heterosexual males to determine if the Centerfold Syndrome could be supported with data. They found that past exposure to pornography was correlated to all five elements of the Centerfold Syndrome. Recent exposure to pornography was also related to increases in sexual reductionism, masculinity validation, and nonrelational sex beliefs for males who view less pornography than their peers. The researchers found that these effects persisted for approximately two days after exposure.

While there are still questions about the validity of the Centerfold Syndrome, the five beliefs that are identified in the theory are also identified in much of the other research examining adolescent consumption of SEIM and attitudes or beliefs. What follows is a review of some pertinent literature about these issues. Peter and Valkenburg (2016) offer a means of categorizing the research as that

32 *Thoughts and values*

which is related to *permissive sexual attitudes*, *gender-specific sexual beliefs*, and *sexual self-development*.

Permissive sexual attitudes

A number of research studies have examined relationships between adolescents' use of SEIM and their attitudes about sex and sexuality. For the purpose of this discussion, *permissive sexual attitudes* refer to positive beliefs about having casual sex, usually outside a romantic relationship or in an uncommitted relationship. It is important to note that in many of the studies, adolescents typically rejected permissive sexual attitudes. In other words, generally speaking, young people do not have a propensity toward believing that casual sex is something they want (Peter & Valkenburg, 2016).

That said, there is research that suggests relationships exist between adolescent consumption of SEIM and permissive attitudes toward sex. Peter and Valkenburg (2008a) sampled 2,343 Dutch adolescents to examine relationships between sexual media consumption and their attitudes toward sex. The authors found that as consumption of sexualized media increased, so did permissive sexual attitudes. Specifically, the study examined attitudes toward sexual relationships with friends, or other casual partners, or in engaging in one-night stands.

Brown and L'Engle (2009) examined the relationship between SEIM and sexual norms among U.S. adolescents. Specifically, the study examined sexual norms using the Personal Sexual Norms Scale created by Sprecher, McKinney, and Orbuch (1991). This scale examines attitudes, such as whether someone should engage in sexual intercourse before marriage or if premarital sex is acceptable if the people are in love. The authors found that as SEIM consumption increased among adolescents, their sexual norms were more progressive, as measured by the instrument (Brown & L'Engle, 2009).

Building on previous research, one study sought to examine how permissive sexual norms develop over time and with relation to SEIM consumption among Dutch teenagers (Doornwaard, Van den Eijnden, Overbeek, & ter Bogt, 2015). The trajectories found in the study suggest that adolescent boys were more likely to use SEIM over time and that their sexual attitudes also became more progressive over that same period. The study found the opposite to be true for girls; that is, over time, girls' sexual attitudes did not become more permissive. In fact, the authors found that girls' SEIM use was consistently low and that their permissive sexual attitudes decreased over time (Doornwaard et al., 2015).

In another study by Peter and Valkenburg (2006), the researchers sought to find connections between the perceived realism of SEIM and teenagers' attitudes toward sex. In examining the survey results of 471 adolescents, the researchers found that males perceived SEIM to be more realistic than did their female peers. They also found that as the subjects' perceived realism increased, so did their permissive sexual attitudes. In short, the study suggests that gender is an important element of this relationship, but when adolescents perceive SEIM to be realistic, their attitudes about sexuality become more permissive.

Lo and Wei (2005) found that exposure to SEIM had a positive relationship with the development of permissive sexual attitudes among Taiwanese adolescents, and Braun-Courville and Rojas (2009) found similar results in a study of U.S. teenagers. In the latter study, the authors examined a number of sexual values, such as emotional commitment, casual sex, one-night stands, and having multiple sexual partners. The study also examined issues of birth control and who bears responsibility for safer sex practices, emotional connection between sexual partners, and purpose of sexual behavior. The authors found a number of correlations between consumption of SEIM and progressive sexual attitudes.

The research leaves the helping professional to consider the relationships between adolescent SEIM consumption and attitudes toward sexual behavior. If these studies are an accurate reflection of reality, then helping professionals should take note. Adolescents will consume SEIM, of that we can be sure. But what about the impact on permissive sexual attitudes? Are these attitudes healthy for a developing teenager? As these attitudes toward sexual permissiveness develop, what, if any, impact will they have on sexual behavior?

As noted at the opening of this section, generally speaking, adolescent attitudes toward sexual permissiveness are low; many teens are not interested in engaging in casual sex, having sex with multiple partners, or having sex outside of a committed relationship. As such, the findings here should be considered with some degree of caution. However, we do know that adolescence is a time of significant development, cognitively and affectively. As teens begin to develop their own values around sex and sexuality, how does their consumption of SEIM influence this development? As helping professionals, do we have an obligation to intervene in these issues? We will discuss intervention approaches later in this chapter, but for now, we encourage the reader to consider how helping professionals might approach these questions through Learning Activity 3.1.

Learning Activity 3.1

I didn't come here to talk about porn

The intention of this exercise is to challenge you to consider how you might use some of the research about sexually permissive attitudes in your work as a helper. Read the case vignette and consider the questions that follow:

Kathryn is a 16-year-old straight female who has presented to counseling with concerns related to depression and anxiety. In one session, Kathryn discloses that while she is not sexually active or in a relationship, she is attracted to a boy in her class named Ben. She has tried flirting with him, and Ben has shown a genuine interest in her, but she's not sure if that interest is sexual or romantic. She is sure Ben is sexually active, as he has dated one of Kathryn's acquaintances, and she's heard talk of their sexual activity.

Kathryn shares with you in session that she's sure Ben would want to be sexually active in any relationship, and she's not sure if she should pursue a romantic relationship or just casual sex. Kathryn shares that while she's "a virgin, she has fooled around with boys before. It's not a big deal." She tells you that she assumes that if she and Ben will be in a relationship that she'll "need to have sex with him; that's just how it is."

Having read the research in this chapter, as her counselor, you think that perhaps her permissive sexual attitudes are related to SEIM consumption.

"So I have to ask you," you begin, "do you ever view pornography?"

"WHAT?!?!" Kathryn yells. "Why on earth would you ask me THAT? What does that have to do with anything we're talking about?"

Consider the following questions:

1. Was this an appropriate question? Why or why not? Consider the purpose behind the question and the pros and cons of the research around this topic.
2. What type of information could this question illicit from Kathryn?
3. What could this helper do to move this discussion forward?
4. Is there a different way the helper could gather the data he or she is seeking? What is the purpose of finding the answer to this question?

Gender-stereotypical sexual beliefs

A cross-section of the research has focused on the relationships between adolescent SEIM consumption and stereotypical gender attitudes and beliefs. The term *gender-stereotypical sexual belief* refers to the notion that "traditional, stereotypical notions of male and female roles as well as of other gender relations dominate" (Peter & Valkenburg, 2016, p. 519). In these research studies, the authors sought to determine if relationships exist between adolescent consumption of SEIM and assumptions about males and females, as well as the objectification of females as sexual objects. Peter and Valkenburg (2009a) define the idea of sex object as "ideas about females that reduce them to their sexual appeal in terms of their outer appearance and their body (parts)" (p. 408).

The portrayal of gender roles in a sexualized society can include either positive themes of intimacy or negative themes of dominant males and submissive females (Moyano & Sierra, 2014). There are also both positive and negative connotations that are associated with the sexual activity in which one engages, but that too depends on one's gender (Ward, Epstein, Caruthers, & Merriwether, 2011). Traditionally, females tend to have more restrictions than their male counterparts in relation to their sexual expression. Consider a teenage male who has multiple sexual partners. Many cultures would allow, or even encourage, the man to brag about his multiple sexual escapades, and he would be elevated by his peers for his desirable deeds. On the other hand, a female who has had multiple sexual partners may find a very different reaction. She might be shamed for her behavior, called a "slut" or a "whore." These are important considerations as the reader examines the overview of the research in this area.

Brown and L'Engle (2009) conducted a student examining 967 young adolescents in the United States. They found that as consumption of SEIM increased, so did stereotypical attitudes about gender. For example, they found correlations between SEIM use and beliefs about gender roles in sports, beliefs about how males and females should act, and whether males should be available for sex more frequently. Peter and Valkenburg (2009a) conducted a similar study that sought to examine a causal relationship between adolescent consumption of SEIM and notions of females as sexual objects. That is, their research study did not simply examine a correlation between these variables but instead examined if consumption of SEIM caused a shift in attitude or belief about men's perceptions of females.

Their study found a reciprocal relationship between these two variables or, as they note in the study, "adolescents' exposure to SEIM was both a cause and a consequence of their beliefs that females are sex objects" (Peter & Valkenburg, 2009a, p. 425). They also found that "such notions also entail a strong concern with females' sexual activities as a main criterion of their sexual attractiveness and focus on females as sexual playthings that are eager to fulfill male sexual desires" (p. 408). While the findings are striking and significant, it is also important to note that the authors did not find significant differences between male and female adolescents in this regard. In other words, teenage girls were more likely to view themselves as sexual objects as their SEIM consumption increased.

This study built on work the authors had previous done that examined if there exists a hierarchical structure to adolescent pornography use and if that hierarchy had an impact on the perception of females as sex objects (Peter & Valkenburg, 2007). Specifically, the authors suggested that a hierarchy exists in pornography consumption, from visual images (i.e., pictures) to audio-visual images (i.e., movies, videos). In this study, the authors found that the only significant relationship between pornography consumption and the perception of females as sex objects existed for audio-visual images; the authors found no gender differences between the 745 Dutch males and females in the study (Peter & Valkenburg, 2007).

Another study examined the relationship between media, in general, and attitudes toward gender (ter Bogt, T., Engels, Bogers, & Kloosterman, 2010). In this study of 480 young adolescents in the Netherlands, the researchers found that the relationships between media use and gender stereotypes were strongest for boys. They also found the strongest relationship among all media types existed for Internet use. Some examples of stereotypical statements used in the study included,

> Boys are always ready and willing for sex; they think about it all the time. . . . Girls should really take care of their appearance, boys don't want an ugly girl as a girlfriend. . . . A girl has to look sexy in order to be attractive to boys.
> (ter Bogt et al., 2010, p. 850)

Pornography tends to place an emphasis on females and their bodies and portrays them in degrading ways (Flood, 2007). For example, pornography focuses on the general understanding that females will want sex from males at any time and in anyway the males want. It also depicts females being coerced into sex with a little stimulation or a little force. As we consider this common portrayal, it is important to consider what this means for the adolescents with whom we work. If the depiction is generalizable to the adolescent who may be sitting in our therapy office or medical clinic, then as helpers, we should take note. There is certainly a logic, albeit a concerning one, to the notion that as developing adolescent boys consume pornography, they are more likely to perceive females as sexual objects who are to be valued for their attractiveness and their willingness to engage in sex. While these are attitudes that most in our professions would want to challenge, there is an intuitive nature to these research findings.

What may not be as obvious to us, however, are the findings related to adolescent females. Many of these studies found little or no significant differences between males and females when considering the correlation between SEIM consumption and the perception of females as sex objects. As we think about our work with adolescent females, issues of self-esteem, personal agency, and self-worth are important and are raised often in the therapeutic process. If these studies accurately represent the attitudes of adolescent girls, then it is especially important that we take note. While healthy sexuality is important, perceiving oneself as a sex object would seem contradictory to the ideal of healthy sexual development. If a sex object is the reduction of a person to a collection of body parts that are perceived as attractive, appealing, and useful mainly for sexual gratification, then as helpers, we must be cognizant of how we can encourage both young females and young males to challenge these notions and help young females develop a healthier sense of self that includes greater esteem and agency.

Sexual self-development

The term *sexual self-development* refers to the aspects and tasks adolescents attempt to complete that are related to the development of their sexual selves (Peter & Valkenburg, 2016). Some studies suggest that consumption of SEIM may be related to sexual uncertainty and the extent to which young people are confused or unclear about their sexual attitudes and beliefs (Peter & Valkenburg, 2008a, 2010). This uncertainty may result from a dissonance created during a time of rapid developmental growth and changing value systems. During adolescence, young people are challenged with navigating the differences between the beliefs instilled by family, school, and other adult caregivers with those from other sources; SEIM can be one of those conflicting sources of information that create dissonance for this population.

One area of study is how consumption of SEIM can cause concerns about one's body or sexual performance. A study of 188 college-aged males in Canada examined relationships between consumption of pornography and sexual perceptions of oneself (Morrison, Ellis, Morrison, Bearden, & Harriman, 2007). Specifically, the authors sought to find relationships between SEIM consumption and body esteem (i.e., negative beliefs about one's body and how it is perceived), genital esteem (i.e., negative beliefs about one's genitals, such as length, appearance, and circumference), and sexual esteem (i.e., negative beliefs about one's sexual performance with partners). While the authors did not determine a relationship between pornography consumption and body esteem, they did find relationships with genital esteem and sexual esteem (Morrison et al., 2007). The findings suggest that when young males consume pornography, they are provided with messages about how one is supposed to perform with their partners and that their genitals should resemble what they see in those media. As we know, much of what we see in the media is unrealistic, and the pornographic film stars' appearance and performance are often not necessarily representative of the general public.

Another study examined this topic further. This research examined the relationship between the consumption of SEIM and sexual satisfaction among adolescents (Peter & Valkenburg, 2009b). The authors argue that "sexually explicit material tends to depict exaggerated portrayals of sexual activities and performances" (Peter & Valkenburg, 2009b, p. 172), but adolescents lack the experience to make sense of what they see or put those portrayals into a real-life context. In this study of over 1,000 adolescents, the authors found that as consumption of SEIM increased, satisfaction with one's sexual experiences decreased. The authors also found that for those with less sexual experience, their dissatisfaction was stronger, but they found no differences between the males and females in the study.

Tsitsika et al. (2009) conducted a similar study of Greek adolescents and found that those exposed to SEIM can develop "unrealistic attitudes about sex and misleading attitudes toward relationships" (p. 549). A different research project examined how adolescents may perceive SEIM as something that depicts realistic sexual experiences and its utility for adolescents. Peter and Valkenburg (2010) found that as SEIM use increased among this population, so did "the extent to which the content of SEIM is perceived to be similar to real world sex" (p. 376–377) and an increase in the perception that SEIM is somehow applicable to the real world of sexual intercourse.

Another study examined potential causality between sexualized media and sexual preoccupancy – that is, "a strong cognitive engagement in sexual issues, sometimes at the exclusion of other thoughts" (Peter & Valkenburg, 2008b, p. 208). While sexual curiosity is a normal element of adolescent development, the authors sought to determine if sexualized media would have a greater impact on the attention adolescents pay to sexual thoughts. In the study, the authors examined the sexual preoccupancy of 962 Dutch adolescents. They found that as exposure to sexualized media increased, so did sexual preoccupancy; there was no difference found between the males and females in the study (Peter & Valkenburg, 2008b).

As we consider the implications of these studies for our practice, the findings may prove valuable. As we consider preoccupancy, we may want to consider that both adolescent males and females may become more preoccupied with sexual thoughts as their consumption of SEIM increases. While it is widely assumed that adolescents can be preoccupied with sexual thoughts, does an increase in this preoccupancy pose any concerns? If thoughts of sex become more common than for peers who consume less SEIM, are there potential consequences academically, socially, or occupationally?

Cognitive dissonance is a common experience in adolescence. Cognitive development is expanding at a rapid pace, and teenagers are exposed to a variety of messages about a multitude of different topics. Information comes from school, peers, television, the Internet, and every other corner of society. These messages may differ from those previously instilled by family, school, and other adult sources. Dissonance is always challenging, but when that dissonance is related to one's sexuality, a topic that is taboo to discuss in many cultures and families, the conflicting messages may become even more challenging to reconcile. What we know about dissonance is that it can be directly related to emotional, behavioral, and cognitive difficulties. It is also common to try to resolve that dissonance as quickly and efficiently as possible to avoid the accompanying discomfort.

There is one other important point in this area of the research related to the needs of adolescent men. As females may receive messages from SEIM that they can be reduced to sexual objects, adolescent males may receive a similar message. If teenage boys compare themselves to the adult pornographic film stars they see in the media, they may consider themselves inadequate. Adolescence is a period of struggle with a sense of inferiority and comparison with others. If teenage boys are comparing themselves to other males who are literally paid to be physically attractive and sexually prosperous, their esteem can certainly suffer as a result.

From theory to practice

As we consider how best to apply the research to our work as helpers, it is important to be discerning with regard to these data. First, this is a sample of studies that have been done in the area of adolescent SEIM consumption and attitudes and beliefs. Each of the studies has its own limitations and considerations. When we consider what is "significant" in quantitative research, we consider effect sizes, p-values (i.e., the probability of obtaining an effect equal to or greater than that found in the sample data), sampling error, and a host of other issues related to research methodology.

Additionally, all research has some implicit bias. While the studies selected were chosen, in part, due to their robust nature, every researcher begins a study with assumptions and expectations; preventing those from biasing one's work is challenging. Related to bias, there are not many researchers examining these issues, so many of the studies are either conducted by the same authors or build on the work of those same researchers. Additionally, as we consider the notion of generalizability, or how relatable the research findings are to the populations with which we each work, we must consider issues of culture. Many of these studies were conducted in Europe or the United States, suggesting a particular bias toward Western culture. Within this Western culture, there are significant differences in attitudes about adolescent sexuality between the many countries where research has been conducted.

Also, there is research in the literature that does point to findings different than those discussed previously. For example, a qualitative study conducted by Löfgren-Mårtenson and Månsson (2010) contradicts some of these findings about permissive sexual attitudes. In this study of 51 Dutch adolescents, the data indicated that the majority of those participants were able to recognize that pornography is largely fantasy, and they were able to distinguish between the depiction of fantasy in pornography and real-life sexual experiences. However, the researchers did find that the messages portrayed in pornographic material do have some influence on teenagers, but as a qualitative study, this research lacks the robust generalizability of a large-sample quantitative study. Still, it is worth consideration as a counterpoint to the research presented previously.

Additionally, some research has suggested that consumption of SEIM may be a normative experience. These studies suggest that consuming pornography may be one element of a normal sexual developmental trajectory and may not have any significant adverse results (Sabina, Wolak, & Finkelhor, 2008; Svedin, Åkerman, & Prieve, 2011; Ybarra & Mitchell, 2005). In one such study of adolescents in the United States, Carroll and associates (2008) found that 67% of adolescent males and 49% of females agreed that consuming pornography was a healthy and normative way of expressing oneself sexually. Löfgren-Mårtenson and Månsson (2010) have argued that SEIM has been normalized culturally in recent years, that society's perspective of pornography has shifted from something that was once "regarded as shameful or morally reprehensible to something socially accepted" (p. 576). In their research, Löfgren-Mårtenson and Månsson (2010) found that adolescents' attitudes about pornography differed greatly depending on their own opinions about sex, gender, and relationships.

Approaches to intervention

The topics discussed in this chapter are difficult to address because they relate to core values that each person holds. Attitudes and beliefs are difficult to address in a helping relationship for a host of reasons. First, they are not obvious. Behaviors can be seen and often have consequences. Behaviors lead to discussion and discussion provides opportunity for intervention. Conversely, attitudes, beliefs, and values are not visible. They may manifest themselves in behavior but are not observable in and of themselves. Additionally, learning about someone's attitudes and beliefs about any topic requires asking the right questions. As we consider the secretive aspects of sexuality, and the taboo nature of discussing sex in some cultures, discovering the attitudes and beliefs that adolescents hold can be a challenging task.

One consideration in approaching attitudes and beliefs is to consider the theoretical approach that one might use from a counseling perspective. Cognitive-behavioral approaches may be appropriate for this type of intervention because they address both thoughts and the behaviors that result from those cognitions. If an adolescent is engaging in a behavior that is unsafe, unhealthy, or otherwise concerning, the helper can ask about the thoughts that client has about him or herself, the world, and his or her own behaviors. For example, if an adolescent client is referred to counseling because his parents are concerned about his promiscuous behavior, the counselor may be able to use those behaviors as an invitation to ask about attitudes. An example might include a question about how the client perceives sexual permissiveness. The client may share that he thinks casual sex is acceptable, which may lead to further discussion about where these beliefs originated. Whether the cognition is a direct result of consumption of SEIM or not, these are still important questions in the therapeutic process.

The research literature also provides some intervention considerations worthy of note. Many of the authors of these studies suggest that improved sexual education is critical when addressing the relationship between the consumption of pornography and the attitudes and beliefs of adolescents. Peter and Valkenburg (2009b) point out that there are concerning findings in the Netherlands regarding consumption of SEIM and the perception of females as sex objects. As they explain, "Even in a sexually liberal country with comprehensive sex education, such as The Netherlands, adolescents are not uniformly educated about the social and sexual reality they may encounter in SEIM" (Peter and Valkenburg, 2009b p. 428). One might consider the effects in countries with more conservative attitudes toward sex and less comprehensive sexual education.

What Peter and Valkenburg (2009b) make clear is that sexual education should also include education about the nature of the messages depicted in SEIM and other pornographic material. Sexual education is often limited to issues related to biology, contraception, sexually transmitted infections, and safer sex methods. However, these topics do not begin to approach a discussion of SEIM. What may be called for are discussion about healthy relationships and the introduction of physical intimacy in relationships. While we may educate adolescents about the physical risks of one-night stands (e.g., sexually transmitted infections, sexual assault), we often do not educate on the emotional risks and potential consequences. At an age when impulsivity is the norm, these are messages that could very well make a difference.

While we may consider how sexual education could be implemented by our schools, that may be a tall order. For school counselors or school psychologists, there may be a need for advocacy around comprehensive sexual education that addresses these issues. Using the research findings discussed here and throughout the literature may prove important in creating empirical support for such advocacy efforts. While school systems may be apprehensive to engaging in these types of practices, empirical data may be helpful in generating and sustaining discussion about these issues.

For those in the helping professions, there are many opportunities to engage in this type of psychoeducation outside of systemic curriculum. Any counselor, psychologist, social worker, nurse, or physician can engage their clientele in discussions about healthy sexuality. While those discussions have often focused on the same topics that sexual education programs have (e.g., safer sex, pregnancy), a paradigm shift to relational education may also be warranted. Educating about the reality, or lack thereof, in SEIM and other pornography may prove critical in an adolescent's development. Challenging the notion of the female as a sex object is paramount, for both adolescent males and females. Educating and enabling parents and other caregivers to engage in these discussions as part of their parenting skills could prove remarkable.

To, Kan, and Ngai (2013) examined the impact of parent-child interactions related to SEIM on various outcomes related to attitudes and beliefs. While the study yielded mixed findings across different domains, the authors strongly advocate for more frequent and better-quality interactions between parents and adolescents related to the consumption of SEIM. The authors argue, "Practitioners should expand their focus of intervention on parent-adolescent communication about prevention of possible negative influence from [SEIM] on adolescents" (To et al., 2013, p. 763). They argue that this is especially important in cultures where discussion of sexual issues is taboo and "adolescents are not used to discussing the related topics with their parents" (To et al., 2013, p. 763).

The authors in this study also point to the importance of peer interactions in relation to the development of attitudes and beliefs about sexuality after consuming SEIM. The authors argue that the peer-to-peer interactions have a profound influence on these developing values and beliefs (To et al., 2013). This study found significant effects of peer-group influence related to SEIM consumption and the development of the attitudes and beliefs discussed throughout this chapter. The authors argue that "intervention and education strategies that acknowledge peer effects should also involve the fostering of positive peer support and learning" (To et al., 2013, p. 763). They suggest that group approaches may prove beneficial in mediating these peer-related effects. Groups that are developed in an atmosphere of trust and understanding allow adolescents to share their struggles and challenges with SEIM with their peers (To et al., 2013).

Learning Activity 3.2 invites the reader to consider different intervention strategies that might be used in a school setting to mediate the potential negative effects of SEIM consumption of adolescents' attitudes and beliefs.

Learning Activity 3.2

Developing systemic interventions

Given what you have learned about the possible impact of adolescent consumption of SEIM on attitudes and beliefs, consider what intervention strategies you might want to employ in a high school setting. In this exercise, do not allow yourself to be bound by issues of resources or social taboos. If you were able to implement whatever strategies you thought would be beneficial, what approaches would you take? Consider the following questions:

1. What individual strategies would you implement? What would be the focus? Who would be responsible for implementation?
2. Would you consider group interventions? If so, what factors would you need to create within the group in order for it to be successful (e.g., trust). Who would be best positioned to implement these strategies?
3. Would you want to include family or other caregivers in your interventions? How would you go about doing so?
4. Are there any other systemic influences you would want to address? How would you address these factors?

Conclusion

This chapter examined the relationships between adolescent consumption of SEIM and the development of attitudes and beliefs about sexuality. While attitudes and beliefs cannot be directly correlated with behavior, these are highly important considerations for human services professionals who work with this population. The research suggests that there are strong correlations and, in some cases, even casual relationships between adolescent use of SEIM and the development of sexually permissive attitudes, gender-stereotypical sexual beliefs, and sexual self-development. While these findings do have their limitations, the results are important for helpers to consider as they assist adolescents in navigating the difficult world of healthy sexual development. Recommendations for practice include specific theoretical techniques, as well as systemic approaches, including parents, families, peers, and psychoeducation in schools and other community resources.

Summary

- The Centerfold Syndrome suggests that heterosexual male sexuality is largely driven by media, and the effect that media has on males leads them to objectify females. The five sets of beliefs associated with the Centerfold Syndrome include (1) voyeurism, (2) sexual reductionism, (3) masculinity validation, (4) trophyism, and (5) nonrelational sex.

- The research associated with adolescent SEIM consumption and attitudinal development may be categorized in three ways: *permissive sexual attitudes*, *gender-specific sexual beliefs*, and *sexual self-development*.
- Permissive sexual attitudes refer to positive beliefs about having casual sex, usually outside a romantic relationship or in an uncommitted relationship. A number of studies have found both correlational and causal relationships between SEIM use and these attitudes.
- The term *gender-stereotypical sexual belief* refers to the notion that "traditional, stereotypical notions of male and female roles as well as of other gender relations dominate" (Peter & Valkenburg, 2016, p. 519). Several studies have explored the relationships between SEIM consumption and the perception of females as sex objects, as well as other stereotypical attitudes.
- The term *sexual self-development* refers to the aspects and tasks adolescents attempt to complete that are related to the development of their sexual selves. Studies have examined issues related to preoccupancy with sexual thoughts, sexual esteem issues in young men, sexual uncertainty, confusion around sexual norms, and sexual satisfaction.
- These studies do have limitations related to bias, research methodology, and cultural considerations.
- Intervention approaches can be individual, group based, or systemic. At the core of the interventions suggested in the literature is the importance of psychoeducation, not only on traditional sexual education topics but also education about SEIM and the messages and lack of reality contained in much of these media.

Additional resources

In print

Brooks, G. R. (1995). *The centerfold syndrome*. San Francisco, CA: Jossey-Bass.

Peter, J., & Valkenburg, P. (2016). Adolescents and pornography: A review of 20 years of research. *The Journal of Sex Research*, *53*(4–5), 509–531.

On the web

McCarthy, J. (2010). Over four in 10 in U.S. now say teen sex is morally acceptable. *Gallup*. Retrieved from https://news.gallup.com/poll/235415/four-say-teen-sex-morally-acceptable.aspx

Vrangalova, Z. (2014). Is casual sex on the rise in America? *Psychology Today*. Retrieved from www.psychologytoday.com/us/blog/strictly-casual/201404/is-casual-sex-the-rise-in-america

References

Barbee, A. P. (1997). Troubled men. *Contemporary Psychology*, *42*, 420–421.

Barbee, A. P. (1998). Show me the data. *Contemporary Psychology*, *43*, 230.

Braun-Courville, D. K., & Rojas, M. (2009). Exposure to sexually explicit web sites and adolescent sexual attitudes and behaviors. *Journal of Adolescent Health*, *45*, 156–162. doi:10.1016/j.jadohealth.2008.12.004

Brooks, G. R. (1995). *The centerfold syndrome*. San Francisco, CA: Jossey-Bass.
Brown, J. D., & L'Engle, K. L. (2009). X-rated: Sexual attitudes and behaviors associated with U.S. early adolescents' exposure to sexually explicit media. *Communication Research, 36*(1), 129–151. doi:10.1177/0093650208326465
Carroll, J., Padilla-Walker, L., Nelson, L., Olson, C., Barry, C., & Madsen, S. (2008). Generation XXX: Pornography acceptance and use among emerging adults. *Journal of Adolescent Research, 23*(1), 6–30. doi:10.1177/0743558407306348
Doornwaard, S., Van den Eijnden, R., Overbeek, G., & ter Bogt, T. (2015). Differential developmental profiles of adolescents using sexually explicit internet material. *Journal of Sex Research, 52*(3), 269–281. doi:10.1080/00224499.2013.866195
Flood, M. (2007). Exposure to pornography among youth in Australia. *Journal of Sociology, 43*, 45–60. doi:10.1177/1440783307073934
Lo, V., & Wei, R. (2005). Exposure to Internet pornography and Taiwanese adolescents' sexual attitudes and behavior. *Journal of Broadcasting and Electronic Media, 49*(2), 221–237. doi:10.1207/s15506878jobem4902_5
Löfgren-Mårtenson, L., & Månsson, S. (2010). Lust, love, and life: A qualitative study of Swedish adolescents' perceptions and experiences with pornography. *Journal of Sex Research, 47*, 568–579. doi:10.1080/00224490903151374
Morrison, T. G., Ellis, S. R., Morrison, M. A., Bearden, A., & Harriman, R. L. (2007). Exposure to sexually explicit material and variations in body esteem, genital attitudes, and sexual esteem among a sample of Canadian men. *The Journal of Men's Studies, 14*(2), 209–222. doi:10.3149/jms.1402.209
Moyano, N., & Sierra, J. C. (2014). Positive and negative sexual cognitions: Similarities and differences between males and women from southern Spain. *Sexual and Relationship Therapy, 29*(4), 454–466. doi:10.1080/14681994.2014.934667
Peter, J., & Valkenburg, P. M. (2006). Adolescents' exposure to sexually explicit online material and recreational attitudes toward sex. *Journal of Communication, 56*(4), 639–660. doi:10.1111/j.1460-2466.2006.00313.x
Peter, J., & Valkenburg, P. M. (2007). Adolescents' exposure to a sexualized media environment and their notions of women as sex objects. *Sex Roles, 56*(5), 381–395. doi:10.1007/s11199-006-9176-y
Peter, J., & Valkenburg, P. M. (2008a). Adolescents' exposure to sexually explicit Internet material, sexual uncertainty, and attitudes toward uncommitted sexual exploration: Is there a link? *Communication Research, 35*(5), 579–601. doi:10.1177/0093650208321754
Peter, J., & Valkenburg, P. M. (2008b). Adolescents' exposure to sexually explicit Internet material and sexual preoccupancy: A three-wave panel study. *Media Psychology, 11*(2), 207–234. doi:10.1080/15213260801994238
Peter, J., & Valkenburg, P. M. (2009a). Adolescents' exposure to sexually explicit Internet material and notions of women as sex objects: Assessing causality and underlying processes. *Journal of Communication, 59*(3), 407–433. doi:10.1111/j.1460-2466.2009.01422.x
Peter, J., & Valkenburg, P. M. (2009b). Adolescents' exposure to sexually explicit Internet material and sexual satisfaction: A longitudinal study. *Human Communication Research, 35*(2), 171–194. doi:10.1111/j.1468-2958.2009.01343.x
Peter, J., & Valkenburg, P. M. (2010). Adolescents' use of sexually explicit Internet material and sexual uncertainty: The role of involvement and gender. *Communication Monographs, 77*(3), 357–375. doi:10.1080/03637751.2010.498791
Peter, J., & Valkenburg, P. M. (2016). Adolescents and pornography: A review of 20 years of research. *The Journal of Sex Research, 53*(4–5), 509–531. doi:10.1080/00224499.2016.1143441

Sabina, C., Wolak, J., & Finkelhor, D. (2008). The nature and dynamics of Internet pornography exposure for youth. *CyberPsychology & Behavior, 11*, 691–693. doi:10.1089/cpb.2007.0179

Sprecher, S., McKinney, K., & Orbuch, T. L. (1991). The effect of current sexual-behavior on friendship, dating, and marriage desirability. *Journal of Sex Research, 28*(3), 387–408. doi:10.1080/00224499109551615

Svedin, C. G., Åkerman, I., & Prieve, G. (2011). Frequent users of pornography: A population based epidemiological study of Swedish male adolescents. *Journal of Adolescence, 34*, 779–788. doi:10.1016/j.adolescence.2010.04.010

ter Bogt, T., Engels, F., Bogers, M., & Kloosterman, R. (2010). "Shake it baby, shake it": Media preferences, sexual attitudes and gender stereotypes among adolescents. *Sex Roles, 63*(11), 844–859. doi:10.1007/s11199-010-9815-1

To, S., Kan, S., & Ngain. S. S. (2013). Interaction effects between exposure to explicit online materials and individual, family, and extramarital factors on Hong Kong high school students' beliefs about gender role equality and body-centered sexuality. *Youth and Society, 47*, 747–768. doi:10.1177/0044118X13490764

Tsitsika, A., Critselis, E., Kormas, D., Konstantoulaki, E., Constantopoulos, A., & Kafetzis, D. (2009). Adolescent pornographic Internet site use: A multivariate regression analysis of the predictive factors of use and psychosocial implications. *CyberPsychology and Behavior, 12*, 545–550. doi:10.1089=cpb.2008.0346

Ward, L., Epstein, M., Caruthers, A., & Merriwether, A. (2011). Men's media use, sexual cognitions, and sexual risk behavior: Testing a mediational model. *Developmental Psychology, 47*, 592–602. doi:10.1037/a0022669

Wright, P. J. (2012). Show me the data! Empirical support for the "Centerfold Syndrome". *Psychology of Men & Masculinity, 13*(2), 180–198. doi: 10.1037/a0023783

Wright, P., & Tokunaga, R. (2015). Activating the Centerfold Syndrome: Recency of exposure, sexual explicitness, past exposure to objectifying media. *Communication Research, 42*(6), 864–897. doi:10.1177/0093650213509668

Ybarra, M. L., & Mitchell, K. J. (2005). Exposure to internet pornography among children and adolescents: A national survey. *CyberPsychology and Behavior, 8*, 473–486. doi:10.1089/cpb.2005.8.473

4 From thinking to doing

The impact on behavior and sexual decision making

> As I'm working with teenage clients, I'm seeing adolescents making dangerous decisions when it comes to sex. It's always been that way, I know. Sexual exploration is normal at this age. But I really wonder. They spend so much time online, and they have unlimited access to sexual material on the Internet. On their phones. On their tablets. Even on their gaming systems. I wonder if there is some connection between the sexual behaviors I'm seeing and all of that unlimited access to electronic pornography?

Many researchers have tried to answer the question posed by the clinician in the vignette. As helpers, we see the unfettered access adolescents have to technology and, in turn, the Internet. We also know that SEIM is available widely online. As discussed in the Chapter 1, we know that adolescents are accessing SEIM, but what we struggle to understand is what influence, if any, that access has on behaviors and decision making?

The purpose of this chapter is to examine the research related to this question, as well as offer suggestions to clinicians and other helpers about how to use these findings in their work. We will begin with a caveat about this research that we will repeat throughout the chapter. While these studies may find correlations between SEIM consumption and particular behaviors, we cannot assume that those relationships are causal. That is, none of the studies examined here can argue that consumption of SEIM does or does not *cause* a behavior to occur. Instead, what the research suggests is that there may be correlations between SEIM consumption and behavior. However, the reasons for those behaviors cannot be assumed and may be related to other causes not examined in these studies.

After reading this chapter, you should be able to

1 Appreciate the relationships found in the research between adolescent consumption of SEIM and negative behavioral outcomes;
2 Consider how one's own attitudes and beliefs about SEIM and adolescent sexuality may impact practice as a human service worker; and
3 Develop intervention strategies for individual clients as well as the systems in which they exist.

Sexual experience and casual sex

One area of focus for researchers has been the relationship between the consumption of SEIM and sexual practices and experiences, such as the decision to engage in sexual activity, participation in casual sex, or the age of one's first sexual experience. A number of studies have found that the more frequent the consumption of pornography, the greater likelihood that adolescents will engage in sexual intercourse (Attwood et al., 2011, Bogale & Seme, 2014; Brown & L'Engle, 2009; Manaf et al., 2014). Cheng, Ma, and Missari (2014) found that this association between SEIM and participation in sexual activity was stronger for young females than it was for young males.

In a study of over 2,000 Scottish teenagers, researchers found that those who consumed SEIM with members of the opposite sex were more likely to engage in sexual activity, while this behavior was less likely among those who consumed SEIM with same-sex peers or when parents restricted the consumption of SEIM (Parkes, Wight, Hunt, Henderson, & Sargent, 2013). Another study of 782 heterosexual adolescents found that as SEIM increased, it was more likely that participants would be engaged in sexual activity (Morgan, 2011). A study of approximately 1,600 Dutch adolescents found that engagement with SEIM through social media was correlated with increases in sexual activity, specifically oral and vaginal intercourse (van Oosten, Peter, & Boot, 2014). Villani (2001) conducted a review of ten years of literature between 1991 and 2001 and found that consumption of pornography was correlated with accelerated onset of sexual activity.

Regarding casual sex, a longitudinal study of Taiwanese youth found a correlation between the consumption of SEIM and engagement in casual sex (Cheng et al., 2014). Two other studies of Taiwanese youth found similar results (Lo et al., 1999; Lo & Wei, 2005), as well as one study in Sweden (Mattebo, Tydén, Häggström-Nordin, Nilsson, & Larsson, 2014). Another study examined the relationships between SEIM, sexual use of social media, and participation in casual sex. Researchers found that exposure to SEIM was directly related to a willingness to engage in casual sex, and that engagement with sexually explicit social media was also correlated with casual sexual behavior (van Oosten, Peter, & Vandenbosch, 2017).

Morgan (2011) found a similar relationship between SEIM use and participation in casual sex. In this study, the author also examined if a correlation existed between the consumption of SEIM and the age at which adolescents begin to engage in sexual activity. Morgan (2011) found that frequency of SEIM consumption was directly correlated with younger ages of first sexual intercourse; that is, younger ages of sexual activity follow increased SEIM use. It should be noted that studies have found that males tend to be exposed to SEIM at a younger age than females (Hald, 2006; Johansson & Hammere´n, 2007).

In other studies, Kraus and Russell (2008) found that young males who have access to SEIM reported engaging in oral sex at a younger age, and both adolescent males and females with SEIM access reported engaging in intercourse at a younger age. While the study discussed a number of limitations (e.g., small effect sizes and possible skewed sampling), it does raise important questions about the relationship between SEIM and the age when adolescents first engage in sexual activity.

In a study of Australian youth, researchers sampled 941 young adults regarding their use of SEIM and their age of first sexual intercourse (Lim, Agius, Carrotte, Vella, & Hellard, 2017). The authors found associations between a number of factors and the consumption of SEIM, including a younger age of sexual activity and engagement in anal intercourse. While the authors stress that the study is not causal, they do point out the importance of the correlation found between these factors.

These findings suggest that correlations do exist between the consumption of SEIM and the likelihood of engaging in sexual activity. However, it should be noted that in many studies, it is found that many adolescents do not engage in sexual activity at all, so the increased likelihood is among a smaller portion of this population. As Peter and Valkenburg (2016) point out, "This means that adolescents' pornography use was associated with a low rate of these behaviors rather than with their massive occurrence" (p. 524).

High-risk behavior

Researchers have sought to find relationships between adolescent consumption of SEIM and the practice of high-risk sexual behaviors. Before discussing research findings, a qualification is warranted. The term "high-risk behavior" is a socially modified construct, and there is subjectivity within the literature. For example, the number of sexual partners one engages with might be considered "high risk"; it might not. Additionally, the decision to engage in sexual intercourse for the first time (i.e., losing one's virginity) may be considered risky behavior based on a number of factors, including age, psychosocial development, cultural contexts, and so forth. In this section, we aim to provide an overview of the literature related to some of the behaviors; however, we do so with the aforementioned caution in mind. We allow readers to determine for themselves what constitutes "high-risk" adolescent sexual behavior.

The research that examined correlations between adolescent SEIM consumption and high-risk sexual behavior yielded mixed results (Peter & Valkenburg, 2016). Van Ouytsel, Ponnet, and Walrave (2014) found that as consumption of SEIM increased among adolescents so did the practice of sexting – that is, sending sexually suggestive images of oneself to others. Luder et al. (2011) found that adolescent males who consume SEIM were more likely to have unprotected sex but that this was not true of adolescent females. Conversely, Peter and Valkenburg (2011) found no correlation between SEIM consumption and high-risk sexual behaviors among adolescents. In the Luder et al. (2011) study discussed previously, researchers found no correlation between SEIM consumption and the number of sexual partners or the decision to engage in intercourse before age 15. In another study, researchers found a relationship between adolescent males' use of SEIM and the number of lifetime partners, as well as acceptance of extramarital sexual relationships (Carroll et al., 2008).

Morrison, Bearden, Harriman, Morrison, and Ellis (2004) also examined possible relationships between SEIM consumption and risky sexual behavior. They found positive correlations between SEIM use and the number of sexual partners for females and one's sexual status (i.e., virgin or not a virgin) for both genders. Similarly, Adebayo, Udegbe, and Sunmola (2006) examined the relationship between Internet use and sexuality among adolescents in Nigeria. The researchers found that as adolescent use of the Internet increased so did the frequency of sexual behavior.

Sexual aggression and victimization

The research related to the consumption of SEIM and acts of sexual aggression or violence is also mixed. For example, Bonino, Ciairano, Rabaglietti, and Cattelino (2006) examined SEIM consumption among Italian boys and found no relationship between viewing pornographic films or videos and engagement in sexual harassment or sexual assault. However, Brown and L'Engle (2009) found that as adolescent male consumption of SEIM increased so did the likelihood of sexual harassment among U.S. adolescent men.

Another study examined male adolescents in the United States and the relationship between SEIM and sexual assault (Ybarra, Mitchell, Hamburger, Diener-West, & Leaf, 2011). Researchers found that while there was no significant correlation between consumption of nonviolent SEIM and sexual assault, a correlation did exist between consumption of violent SEIM and in-person sexual violence perpetration. In this study, the researchers also examined the perpetration of sexual violence through technology and found a positive relationship between the consumption of violent SEIM and technology-based sexual harassment (i.e., coercing someone to engage in online sexual behavior with which they were not comfortable).

If the research does suggest the possibility of relationships between SEIM and sexual aggression, the correlate is also worthy of review; that is, is SEIM consumption related to sexual victimization? The study examining Italian adolescents mentioned previously also explored this question. Bonino et al. (2006) found positive relationships between the consumption of sexual videos and films and surviving sexual violence. A study of Chinese youth found a correlation between the consumption of pornography and polyvictimization (i.e., multiple types of abuse, including sexual abuse) among both male and female adolescents (Dong, Cao, Cheng, Cui, & Li, 2013). Finally, a study of Ethiopian adolescents found strong correlations between consumption of pornographic films and sexual victimization among young females (Bekele, Van Aken, & Dubas, 2011).

SEIM and addiction

When we consider the possibility of addiction to SEIM Internet pornography, the majority of adolescent consumers will never experience any problematic behavior or significant negative consequences. For the most part, many youth are simply recreational consumers of Internet pornography, much like someone who "surfs the web." Recreational users are thought to consume Internet pornography as a means of education, stimulation, entertainment, or out of boredom, with little chance of developing any problematic behaviors (Cooper, Griffin-Shelley, Delmonico, & Mathy, 2001). This casual consumption of SEIM does not detract from everyday life, and the vast majority of adolescents will show no signs of obsession or compulsion (Cooper, Delmonico, Griffin-Shelley, & Mathy, 2004). While the potential of developing obsessive or compulsive behaviors is relatively low, there are risks for problematic use of SEIM.

According to the *Diagnostic and Statistical Manual of Mental Disorders*, fifth edition (American Psychiatric Association, 2013), obsessions are defined as "recurrent and persistent thoughts, urges, or impulses that are experienced, at some time during the disturbance, as intrusive and unwanted, and that in most individuals cause marked anxiety or distress" (p. 235). Adolescents who spend a great deal of time thinking about Internet pornography or consuming SEIM may have developed an obsession. For many, an attempt to satisfy such an obsession may become a compulsive behavior. Compulsive behavior is defined as "repetitive behaviors . . . that the individual feels driven to perform in response to an obsession" (American Psychiatric Association, 2013, p. 235). Compulsive consumers of SEIM may demonstrate a preoccupation with Internet pornography (Cooper et al., 2001) and experience an inability to regulate their consumption, which could impact basic everyday life activities (Cooper et al., 2004). Adolescents who experience an irresistible urge or who continuously consume SEIM believing they can stop may have established a compulsive behavior.

It is possible that individuals with an addiction to Internet pornography may experience similar process-related symptoms to that of individuals with substance addictions (Laier, Pekal, & Brand, 2014). For example, individuals who consume alcohol over a period of time will eventually develop a tolerance and need to increase the amount of consumption in order to achieve the desired effect. The same type of tolerance may be applied to the consumption of Internet pornography. For example, consider a recreational user consuming Internet pornography for the purpose of masturbation. Over time, the desired effect of orgasm may not be achieved in a few minutes but perhaps only after a few hours. In this case, a tolerance may have been established. It should be noted, however, that there are also studies that suggest differences exist between biological addiction and SEIM consumption (e.g., Prause, Steele, Staley, Sabatinelli, & Hajcak, 2015).

Adolescents may consume SEIM as a coping mechanism in times of high stress or to seek relief from depression (Cooper et al., 2004) much like social drinkers who consume alcohol to end a difficult workweek or cope with grief. The same comparison to alcohol abuse could be used when accounting for dependence and symptoms of withdrawal. Consider the adolescent who consumes Internet pornography on a daily basis but is immediately forced to abstain from online access for an extended period of time. Similar to substance abuse, symptoms of withdrawal from SEIM might lead an adolescent to experience different emotional responses, such as irritability, sadness, and so forth.

Many psychological struggles can be self-recognized and at times, even self-diagnosed. This holds true in cases of recognizing a potential addiction to Internet pornography. However, it must be noted that although a perceived addiction to Internet pornography may be an accurate self-diagnosis, there is also an extremely high chance that the underlying issue is something else. For example, many who self-diagnose a perceived addiction to SEIM are not addicted at all, but instead only believe that they are. This feeling of addiction tends to exist more commonly in religious individuals (Grubbs, Wilt, Exline, Pargament, & Kraus, 2017).

For adolescents who identify with certain religious belief systems, the consumption of SEIM is believed to be a sinful and immoral act and can be considered a desecration of sacred religious values. These strongly held religious beliefs may lead some young people to not only experience substantial feelings of guilt and shame but also the perception of an addiction to Internet pornography (Grubbs et al., 2017). The research has suggested that religious individuals who consume Internet pornography are at a higher likelihood of perceiving their behavior as an addiction (Bradley, Grubbs, Uzdavines, Exline, & Pargament, 2016).

Given the convenience, accessibility, and immediate availability of SEIM in the digital age, such problematic behaviors may become more prevalent than in the past. The helping professional must understand when the consumption of SEIM is for recreational use or when an adolescent's consumption has become obsessive or compulsive. Having a working understanding of substance use and abuse may also provide the helping professional with additional insight into process-related addictions, such as CIU. Religious beliefs should be given special attention, and helping professionals working with religious individuals must be able to balance the presenting issue of perceived Internet pornography addiction with the potentially underlying real issue of a breakdown in individual morality (Grubbs et al., 2017).

Conduct issues, substance use, and other mental health concerns

Researchers have also examined relationships between adolescent consumption of SEIM and oppositional behavior or conduct concerns. In a study of 529 Greek adolescents, Tsitsika et al. (2009) explored the relationships between frequency of SEIM consumption and conduct issues (i.e., oppositional behaviors, school and community consequences). The researchers found that infrequent SEIM use was not correlated with negative conduct but instead "reflects transient behavior without negative effects on adolescent development" (Tsitsika et al., 2009, p. 549). However, frequent SEIM use was significantly related to conduct concerns, and the authors argue it "is associated with behavioral and social maladjustment among adolescents" (Tsitsika et al., 2009, p. 549).

Efforts have been made to explore relationships between adolescent use of SEIM and substance abuse. Carroll et al. (2008) sought to determine if there were correlations between SEIM consumption and patterns of alcohol consumption. Analyses found that males who did not use pornography engaged in less consumption of alcohol and less binge drinking than men who did consume pornography. The relationship between substance use and SEIM consumption was even more pronounced in young females. Tapert et al. (2001) have also found relationships between sexual behavior and substance abuse. Again, it should be noted that these are correlations and do not indicate that SEIM consumption leads to substance abuse.

Finally, some evidence suggests relationships between adolescent use of SEIM and other mental health concerns. In one study of Swedish SEIM consumers, the authors found relationships between SEIM consumption and depressive symptoms (Svedin, Åkerman, & Priebe (2011). Among young men, SEIM consumption has been found to be correlated to negative affective symptoms, depression, and high stress levels (Tylka, 2015; Levin, Lillis, & Hayes, 2012).

From theory to practice

While the research provides data and findings to support our work with adolescents who consume SEIM, some warnings should be considered with regard to research findings. First, as discussed previously, none of the studies mentioned here suggest causality. The consumption of SEIM does not *cause* unsafe sex practices, early age of sexual intercourse, mental health concerns, substance use, or any other finding from the literature. Instead, there are relationships or correlations between these variables. But correlations should be considered with some hesitance. Although there is a correlation between SEIM and, say, conduct issues, there may be other reasons for those behaviors or a constellation of reasons.

Second, some of the terms in the literature have different operational definitions. For example, pornography is a subjective construct, and there are differences between intentional consumption of SEIM (i.e., seeking it out) and unintentional consumption (e.g., searching for a popular U.S. sporting goods store only to find a very different website). Also, in some studies, pornography may be merely visual images of nudity or partial nudity, while in other studies, it may include graphic video of sexual acts, some of which may be violent in nature.

Also, each study will have its own specific limitations. Some studies may have small sample sizes or low effect sizes. Culture is an issue when considering the generalizability of many of the studies contained in this chapter. For example, human service workers in the United States or United Kingdom may not find the results of studies in the Netherlands or Sweden as applicable to the populations with which they work. These countries are generally known for more liberal attitudes toward adolescent sexuality and pornography consumption (Peter & Valkenburg, 2016).

In a systematic review of literature related to this topic, Peter and Valkenburg (2016) found that 66% of the studies reviewed focused on adolescents in Europe, North America, or Australia. Also, much of the research lacks the context of normal human development (Peter & Valkenburg, 2016). We know that adolescence is a period of rapid and significant cognitive, emotional, physical, and social change. Most of the studies described here lack consideration of how those changes impact adolescents' use of SEIM and the resulting findings in the research.

Another limitation in the literature reviewed here is related to heteronormative bias. Very few studies examine relationships between SEIM and the behaviors of youth who identify as members of the LGBTQA+ community. Additionally, a negativity bias appears within the literature on adolescent use of SEIM (Peter & Valkenburg, 2016). The research mainly focuses on the potential negative outcomes related to adolescents' consumption of SEIM rather than potential benefits. For example, SEIM may provide adolescents with sexual pleasure. Additionally, while many of these studies attempted to find correlations between multiple variables, only those that were statistically significant are typically reported. As an example, a researcher may be seeking to find relationships between SEIM use and a host of behaviors, such as drug use, conduct issues, age of first sexual experience, and use of safer sex practices. If the data only point to one negative behavioral outcome, say drug use, then it is reported that a correlation exists between SEIM and drug use. However, it is not typically reported that there is also no relationship between SEIM and those other variables. Many researchers simply report that the results were insignificant.

Finally, as mentioned previously in this chapter, there are the biases that we all hold. Those who conduct research possess bias that is difficult to remove from their research work. What constitutes "unsafe sex?" While many may agree that sex without a condom or other barrier device is unsafe, others may argue that any sexual activity between adolescents would be unsafe. What is the age when it is developmentally appropriate to engage in sexual behavior? Certainly, the answer to that question is subjective, and that subjectivity results from a variety of factors, such as value judgments, spiritual beliefs, and family of origin, to name a few.

As you consider how to use these findings in your practice, we encourage you to consider your own biases when it comes to sexuality and adolescents. If a client discloses that he or she is engaged in sexual activity at age 15, is that risky behavior? What if the client is using safer sex methods? What if it is only oral sex as opposed to vaginal or anal sex? Does the client's developmental age play a role in your own value assessment?

Sexuality, especially when considering adolescents, is a highly charged and very personal issue. As a human service professional, it is impossible to remove yourself from your own opinions. However helpers have a responsibility to set their own values, judgments, and morality aside for the benefit of their clients; it is not only good practice, but for many professions, it is an ethical obligation. For example, the American Counseling Association's (ACA) *Code of Ethics* makes it clear that "counselors are aware of – and avoid imposing – their own values, attitudes, beliefs and behaviors" (ACA, 2014, Standard A.4.b.). In Learning Activity 4.1, we encourage readers to consider their own biases and how they can best address them when working with adolescents.

Learning Activity 4.1

Examining our own biases about adolescent sexuality

You have now had an opportunity to review the literature related to SEIM consumption and adolescent behavior. As you think about what you've read, consider the following questions:

1 How would you define sexual behavior? Does your definition include masturbation, oral sex, vaginal sex, anal sex?
2 Do you believe adolescents should be engaging in sexual behavior? At what age do you believe it is appropriate for this population to begin engaging in this behavior?
3 How do you define "risky sexual behavior?"
4 What is an appropriate number of sexual partners for an adolescent, considering the biological and developmental age of the person?
5 What are your opinions about sexual development in adolescence?
6 If you are working directly with an adolescent (or his or her family/caregivers) who holds different views from yours, how will you address this? How can you ensure that you are not imposing your views or values on that client? Is that important to you? Is it an ethical expectation given your profession?

Approaches to intervention

While the research suggests a number of different correlations between adolescent consumption of SEIM and various behaviors, there is scant evidence on how best to intervene with these concerns. The research typically stops short of intervention strategies, in part because many of the studies are exploratory or have yielded mixed results. This leaves the practicing human services worker without clear direction about how best to work with the behaviors that might be results of SEIM consumption.

One approach is to treat the behaviors themselves. For example, if a client is engaged in substance abuse, there are a host of techniques that have empirical support in addressing substance use and abuse in adolescents and young adults (e.g., motivational interviewing or cognitive-behavioral approaches). For conduct concerns, behavioral approaches might be indicated. For adolescents who have found themselves as survivors of violence or sexual harassment, trauma-informed techniques and theories might be helpful (e.g., trauma-focused, cognitive-behavioral therapy, cognitive processing therapy, stress inoculation techniques).

One finding in the literature that may be valuable to counselors and other helpers is the notion that adolescents may use SEIM as a form of sexual education (Perrin et al., 2008; Tsitsika et al., 2009). As discussed previously, adolescence is a time of rapid growth, including sexual development. Curiosity is a normal part of this developmental process, as is the emergence of a sexual self. Tsitsika and associates (2009) found that frequent use of SEIM was correlated with increased visiting of sexual education websites.

This finding suggests that psychoeducation may be an important intervention strategy when working with adolescents and their consumption of SEIM. Wallmyr and Welin (2006) argue that sexual education is critical for adolescents; they found that their sample most often received sexual education from peers and that female adolescents consumed SEIM out of "curiosity" (Wallmyr & Welin, 2006). The authors argue that sex education is important to "give factual information about sexuality to counteract the messages about sexuality presented in pornography" (Wallmyr & Welin, 2006, p. 295).

This begs the question, what can counselors or other helping professionals do to provide this sexual education to clients? One approach for those who work directly with adolescents is to be sure that they themselves are well informed about issues related to sexuality, such as laws related to consent, resources for survivors of sexual assault or harassment, information on sexually transmitted infections, and safer sex methods. Providing sexual psychoeducation during individual or group counseling sessions is critical to ensuring that clients are informed about risks, ways of staying safe, and other information related to adolescent sexuality. Counselors may also want to consider couples-based interventions to open a mature and healthy dialogue between adolescents who are sexually active.

Those who work in settings with large adolescent populations (e.g., school counselors, school psychologists, university counseling staff) may consider large-scale psychoeducation methods. For example, college campuses have long had psychoeducation strategies for informing young adults about risks related to sexual assault, sexually transmitted infections, and safer sex practices. Counselors in these settings may not have as much to do in terms of developing these programs, but continued advocacy for resources and engaging other campus stakeholders are critical to their continued success.

Public school systems in the United States and elsewhere may not have resources available to students at younger ages. In the United States, school-based curricula are largely set by local and state governments, providing for a system where sexual education may differ depending on the norms of a particular local community. In areas where adequate sexual education is lacking, school counselors may choose to advocate for more comprehensive sexual education programs in middle and high schools. They may need to challenge the status quo to ensure that their clientele is adequately educated about issues related to adolescent sexuality. While the consumption of pornography is a complicated and morally charged issue, we believe that many can agree with Wallmyr and Welin's (2006) assertion that SEIM may not be the resource we want adolescents using to learn about healthy sexuality, especially given what we do know from the research.

Learning Activity 4.2 invites readers to consider a case study and how they might engage the client in the presented concern.

Learning Activity 4.2

Jane: a case study in adolescent behaviors

This exercise is intended to challenge readers to consider their knowledge, skills, and attitudes toward technology and pornography. Consider the following case example and then respond to the questions that follow.

Jane is a 16-year-old client who presents for counseling with depressive symptoms. As you unpack Jane's presentation, you begin to learn that much of her unhappiness is related to her relationship with her boyfriend, Matthew. Jane feels like Matthew has some very unrealistic expectations about the physical nature of their relationship. Jane shares with you that she "caught" Matthew looking at pornography on his phone and that what she has seen in the pictures and videos is very different from the physical relationship she wants to have. "I don't really think either of us is ready, but we're having sex anyway. We don't use protection; we both know we should, but we don't. No one in those pictures or videos ever does either. Not to say that it's right, but it's just what it is. And we do some things that I know I'm not really interested in . . . you know . . . but he wants to, and it's what you have to do if you're going to be in a relationship."

Consider this case and the following questions:

1   What do you believe Jane's most significant concerns are? What questions would you want to ask to learn more?
2   How could you help Jane better understand what a healthier sexual relationship might look like?
3   What assumptions is Jane making? Are they correct? If you're unsure, how could you help her to find out?
4   How do *you* feel about what Jane has said? Is there anything that bothers you? How would you deal with your own response to Jane's story?

Conclusion

This chapter provided a review of the research examining relationships between adolescent consumption of SEIM and different behavioral outcomes. While findings are mixed and there are limitations in the methods and generalizability of some studies, there are data in the literature that suggest that relationships exist between adolescent use of SEIM and a host of negative behavioral outcomes, including high-risk sexual behavior, aggression and victimization, substance use, and mental health concerns, such as depression. While care should be taken in interpreting these results, there are things that counselors and other helpers can do to address these concerns, most notably engaging in psychoeducation with adolescent clients to ensure that they are exposed to correct and healthy information regarding their own sexual development.

Summary

- A number of studies have found that the more frequent the consumption of pornography, the greater likelihood that adolescents will engage in sexual intercourse.
- Research suggests that among adolescents, correlations exist between the consumption of SEIM and engagement in casual sex.
- Some studies have found correlations between SEIM and the age when adolescents first engage in sexual activity.
- Some studies have found positive relationships between SEIM use and high-risk sexual behavior, although the term "high risk" is subjective and should be considered within one's values framework.
- Some studies have found correlations between SEIM use and sexual aggression and victimization
- Adolescent consumption of SEIM may become problematic and take on compulsive features in an effort to address obsessive thoughts. Helping professionals may want to consider addiction models when pondering these issues.
- Some research has found relationships between SEIM use and alcohol use, conduct concerns, and mental health issues.
- In translating theory to practice, helpers should be aware of their own values, judgments, and attitudes about SEIM and adolescent sexuality.
- When engaging in intervention, education is critical. Adolescents may seek out SEIM as a means of filling perceived gaps in their own knowledge about sexuality and development. When those messages are provided by trained professionals, we can have more confidence that the information adolescents receive is accurate and healthy.

Additional resources

In print

Buckinham, D., & Bragg, S. (2004). *Young people, sex, and the media: The facts of life?* Basingstoke, UK: Palgrave Macmillan.

Peter, J. (2013). Media and sexual development. In D. Lemish (Ed.), *The Routledge international handbook of children, adolescents, and media* (pp. 217–223). London: Routledge.

Peter, J., & Valkenburg, P. (2016). Adolescents and pornography: A review of 20 years of research. *The Journal of Sex Research*, 53(4–5), 509–531.

On the web

Centers for Disease Control. (n.d.). *CDC Fact Sheet: Information for teens and young adults: Staying healthy and preventing STDs*. Retrieved from www.cdc.gov/std/life-stages-populations/stdfact-teens.htm

Rape, Abuse, and Incest National Network (RAINN). (n.d.). *About RAINN*. Retrieved from www.rainn.org

References

Adebayo, D., Udegbe, I., & Sunmola, A. (2006). Gender, Internet use, and sexual behavior orientation among young Nigerians. *CyberPsychology & Behavior, 9*(6), 742–752. doi:10.1089/cpb.2006.9.742

American Counseling Association. (2014). *2014 ACA code of ethics*. Alexandria, VA: Author.

American Psychiatric Association. (2013). *Diagnostic and statistical manual of mental disorders* (5th ed.). Washington, DC: Author.

Attwood, K. A., Zimmerman, R., Cupp, P. K., Fongkaew, W., Miller, B. A., Bekele, A. B., . . . Dubas, J. S. (2011). Sexual violence victimization among female secondary school students in eastern Ethiopia. *Violence and Victims, 26*(5), 608–630. doi:10.1891/0886-6708.26.5.608

Bekele, A. B., Van Aken, M. A. G., & Dubas, J. S. (2011). Sexual violence victimization among female secondary school students in eastern Ethiopia. *Violence and Victims, 26*, 608–630. doi:10.1891/0886-6708.26.5.608

Bogale, A., & Seme, A. (2014). Premarital sexual practices and its predictors among in-school youths of Shendi town, West Gojjam zone, north western Ethiopia. *Reproductive Health, 11*, 49. doi:10.1186/ 1742-4755-11-49

Bonino, S., Ciairano, S., Rabaglietti, E., & Cattelino, E. (2006). Use of pornography and self-reported engagement in sexual violence among adolescents. *European Journal of Developmental Psychology, 3*(3), 265–288. doi:10.1080/17405620600562359

Bradley, D. E., Grubbs, J. B., Uzdavines, A., Exline, J. J., & Pargament, K. I. (2016). Perceived addiction to Internet pornography among religious believers and non-believers. *Sexual Addiction and Compulsivity, 23*, 225–243. doi:10.1080/10720162.2016.1162237

Brown, J. D., & L'Engle, K. L. (2009). X-rated: Sexual attitudes and behaviors associated with U.S. early adolescents' exposure to sexually explicit media. *Communication Research, 36*(1), 129–151. doi:10.1177/0093650208326465

Carroll, J. S., Padilla-Walker, L. M., Nelson, L. J., Olson, C. D., McNamara Barry, C., & Madsen, S. D. (2008). Generation XXX: Pornography acceptance and use among emerging adults. *Journal of Adolescent Research, 23*(1), 6–30. doi:10.1177/0743558407306348

Cheng, S., Ma, J., & Missari, S. (2014). The effects of Internet use on adolescents' first romantic and sexual relationships in Taiwan. *International Sociology, 29*(4), 324–347. doi:10.1177/0268580914538084

Cooper, A., Delmonico, D. L., Griffin-Shelley, E., & Mathy, R. M. (2004). Sexual Addiction & Compulsivity, *11*(3), 129–143. doi:10.1080/10720160490882642

Cooper, A., Griffin-Shelley, E., Delmonico, D. L., & Mathy, R. M. (2001). Online sexual problems: Assessment and predictive variables. *Sexual Addiction & Compulsivity, 8*, 267–285. doi:10.1080/107201601753459964

Dong, F., Cao, F., Cheng, P., Cui, N., & Li, Y. (2013). Prevalence and associated factors of poly-victimization in Chinese adolescents. *Scandinavian Journal of Psychology, 54*(5), 415–422. doi:10.1111/sjop.12059

Grubbs, J. B., Wilt, J. A., Exline, J. J., Pargament, K. I., & Kraus, S. W. (2017). Moral disapproval and perceived addiction to Internet pornography: A longitudinal study. *Addiction, 113*, 496–506. doi:10.1111/add.14007

Hald, G. M. (2006). Gender differences in pornography consumption among young heterosexual Danish adults. *Archives of Sexual Behavior, 35*, 577–585. doi:10.1007/s10508-006-9064-0

Johansson, T., & Hammere´n, N. (2007). Hegemonic masculinity and pornography: Young people's attitudes toward and relations to pornography. *Journal of Men's Studies, 15*, 57–70. doi:10.3149/jms.1501.57

Kraus, S., & Russell, B. (2008). Early sexual experiences: The role of Internet access and sexually explicit material. *CyberPsychology & Behavior*, *11*(2), 162–168. doi:10.1089/cpb.2007.0054

Laier, C., Pekal, J., & Brand, M. (2014). Cybersex addiction in heterosexual female users of Internet pornography can be explained by gratification hypothesis. *Cyberpsychology, Behavior, and Social Networking*, *17*(8). doi:10.1089/cyber.2013.0396

Levin, M. E., Lillis, J., & Hayes, S. C. (2012). When is online pornography viewing problematic among college males? Examining the moderating role of experiential avoidance. *Sex Addict Compulsivity*, *19*, 168–180. doi:10.1080/10720162.2012.657150

Lim, M., Agius, P., Carrotte, E., Vella, A., & Hellard, M. (2017). Young Australians' use of pornography and associations with sexual risk behaviours. *Australian and New Zealand Journal of Public Health*, *41*(4), 438–443. doi:10.1111/1753-6405.12678

Lo, V., Neilan, E., Sun, M., & Chiang, S. (1999). Exposure of Taiwanese adolescents to pornographic media and its impact on sexual attitudes and behaviour. *Asian Journal of Communication*, *9*(1), 50–71. doi:10.1080/01292989909359614

Lo, V., & Wei, R. (2005). Exposure to Internet pornography and Taiwanese adolescents' sexual attitudes and behavior. *Journal of Broadcasting and Electronic Media*, *49*(2), 221–237. doi:10.1207/s15506878jobem4902_5

Luder, M.-T., Pittet, I., Berchtold, A., Akre, C., Michaud, P. A., & Suris, J. C. (2011). Associations between online pornography and sexual behavior among adolescents: Myth or reality? *Archives of Sexual Behavior*, *40*(5), 1027–1035. doi:10.1007/s10508-010-9714-0

Manaf, M. R. A., Tahir, M. M., Sidi, H., Midin, M., Nik Jaafar, N. R., Das, S., & Malek, A. M. A. (2014). Pre-marital sex and its predicting factors among Malaysian youths. *Comprehensive Psychiatry*, *55*, 82–88. doi:10.1016/j.comppsych.2013.03.008

Mattebo, M., Tydén, T., Häggström-Nordin, E., Nilsson, K. W., & Larsson, M. (2014). Pornography and sexual experiences among high school students in Sweden. *Journal of Developmental & Behavioral Pediatrics*, *35*(3), 179–188. doi:10.1097/DBP.0000000000000034

Morgan, E. (2011). Associations between young adults' use of sexually explicit materials and their sexual preferences, behaviors, and satisfaction. *Journal of Sex Research*, *48*(6), 520–530. doi:10.1080/00224499.2010.543960

Morrison, T. G., Bearden, A., Harriman, R., Morrison, M. A., & Ellis, S. R. (2004). Correlates of exposure to sexually explicit material among Canadian post-secondary students. *The Canadian Journal of Human Sexuality*, *13*(3–4), 143–156. doi:10.3149/jms.1402.209

Parkes, A., Wight, D., Hunt, K., Henderson, M., & Sargent, J. (2013). Are sexual media exposure, parental restrictions on media use and co-viewing TV and DVDs with parents and friends associated with teenagers' early sexual behaviour? *Journal of Adolescence*, *36*(6), 1121–1133. doi:10.1016/j.adolescence.2013.08.019

Perrin, P. C., Madanat, H. N., Barnes, M. D., Carolan, A., Clark, R. B., Ivins, N., & Tuttle, S. R. (2008). Health education's role in framing pornography as a public health issue: Local and national strategies with international implications. *Promotion & Education*, *15*, 11–18. doi:10.1177/1025382307088093

Peter, J., & Valkenburg, P. M. (2011). The influence of sexually explicit Internet material on sexual risk behavior: A comparison of adolescents and adults. *Journal of Health Communication*, *16*(7), 750–765. doi:10.1080/10810730.2011.551996

Peter, J., & Valkenburg, P. M. (2016). Adolescents and pornography: A review of 20 years of research. *The Journal of Sex Research*, *53*(4–5), 509–531. doi:10.1080/00224499.2016.1143441

Prause, N., Steele, V. R., Staley, C., Sabatinelli, D., & Hajcak, G. (2015). Modulation of late positive potentials by sexual images in problem users and controls inconsistent with "porn addiction." *Biological Psychology*, *109*, 192–199. doi:10.1016/j.biopsycho.2015.06.005

Svedin, C. G., Åkerman, I., & Priebe, G. (2011). Frequent users of pornography: A population based epidemiological study of Swedish male adolescents. *Journal of Adolescence*, *34*(4), 779–88. doi:10.1016/j.adolescence.2010.04.010

Tapert, S. E., Aarons, G. A., Sedlar, G. R., & Brown, S. A. (2001). Adolescent substance use and sexual risk-taking behavior. *Journal of Adolescent Health*, *25*(3), 181–189. doi:10.1016/S1054-139X(00)00169-5

Tsitsika, A., Critselis, E., Kormas, G., Konstantoulaki, E., Constantopoulos, A., & Kafetzis, D. (2009). Adolescent pornographic Internet site use: A multivariate regression analysis of the predictive factors of use and psychosocial implications. *CyberPsychology & Behavior*, *12*(5), 545–550. doi:10.1089/cpb.2008.0346

Tylka, T. L. (2015). No harm in looking, right? Men's pornography consumption, body image, and well-being. *Psychology of Men & Masculinity*, *16* (1), 97–107. doi:10.1037/a0035774

van Oosten, J., Peter, J., & Vandenbosch, L. (2017). Adolescents' sexual media use and willingness to engage in casual sex: Differential relations and underlying processes. *Human Communication Research*, *43*(1), 127–147. doi:10.1111/hcre.12098

van Oosten, J., Peter, M., & Boot, F. (2014). Exploring associations between exposure to sexy online self-presentations and adolescents' sexual attitudes and behavior. *Journal of Youth and Adolescence*, *44*(5), 1078–1091. doi:10.1007/s10964-014-0194-8

Van Ouytsel, J., Ponnet, K., & Walrave, M. (2014). The associations between adolescents' consumption of pornography and music videos and their sexting behavior. *Cyberpsychology, Behavior and Social Networking*, *17*(12), 772–778. doi:10.1089/cyber.2014.0365

Villani, S. (2001). Impact of media on children and adolescents: A 10-year review of the research. *Journal of the American Academy of Child and Adolescent Psychiatry*, *40*, 392–401. doi:10.1097/00004583-200104000-00007

Wallmyr, G., & Welin, C. (2006). Young people, pornography, and sexuality: Sources and attitudes. *The Journal of School Nursing*, *22*, 290–295. doi:10.1177/10598405060220050801

Ybarra, M. L., Mitchell, K. J., Hamburger, M., Diener-West, M., & Leaf, P. J. (2011). X-rated material and perpetration of sexually aggressive behavior among children and adolescents: Is there a link? *Aggressive Behavior*, *37*(1), 1–18. doi:10.1002/Ab.20367

5 Thoughts of the self
Pornography and adolescent self-image

I feel horrible for this young male in my practice. He's 15 years old and just got physically intimate with a partner. It's his first time in a sexual relationship, and he seems so lost. He's looking to his partner for some sort of validation, but she's not giving any. I don't even think it's that she doesn't want to, but it's that she doesn't know how. So my client keeps thinking about what he has to do to please her. And if his body is attractive enough for her. If he has a big enough penis. If he is muscular enough. He talks about how he watches pornography on his phone, and he sees the men in those videos and compares himself. But what kind of comparison is that? Those are grown men who got into porn because of certain physical attributes, you know? And here's this young male, a boy really, thinking he needs to measure up? I'm not sure how to tell him he won't, and that should be ok.

The sexualization of human beings across nearly all media is popular for marketing purposes because "sex sells." In many forms of broadcast media, it is likely that one will commonly find actors and actresses who appear physically attractive and who tend to be open and extremely confident in their own sexuality. When we consider SEIM, and pornography as a medium in general, it focuses on nudity, breasts, genitalia, and sexual performance; if one compares themselves to what is depicted in SEIM, sexual standards and expectations increase significantly. However, the increased sexual standards and expectations depicted in Internet pornography are mostly unrealistic and may deviate far from what is considered to be a reasonable standard.

For adolescents in the process of their sexual development, this inaccurate portrayal of sexual reality significantly increases the risk of internalizing such unrealistic expectations. An unhealthy internalization of unrealistic sexual expectations can encourage developing young people to hold themselves to very high and unattainable standards. In addition, extraordinary standards may be expected of their partners. When adolescents aspire to achieve the physical and performance attributes that are depicted in SEIM, they may find themselves adversely affected. For example, youth who internalize Internet pornography may develop body insecurities, feelings of inadequacy, frustration with sexual functioning and performance, and experience overall sexual dissatisfaction. The purpose of this chapter is to give the reader an unbiased overview from a neutral perspective of where Internet pornography intersects with self. As the vignette at the opening of this chapter demonstrates, helping young people navigate these issues can be difficult.

62 *Thoughts of the self*

After reading this chapter, you should be able to

1 Understand how individual body image and social comparisons during youth sexual development can be affected by consumption of SEIM;
2 Know how body image can directly influence sexual satisfaction and sexual self-esteem;
3 Identify how the consumption of Internet pornography can impact self-esteem and overall confidence with individual sexuality;
4 Be knowledgeable of the role SEIM consumption may play in influencing sexual satisfaction and causing sexual dysfunction; and
5 Recognize how Internet pornography may create sexual performance expectations that may be unrealistic.

Self-image and SEIM: understanding the relationships

Through a process of social comparison, many people internalize body image based on the appearance of others. It is not uncommon for adolescents to compare their own bodies, genitals, and sexual performance to that of those idealistic actors found in Internet pornography; this is especially true for young males. For many, this upward comparison may lead to feelings of inadequacy and sexual dissatisfaction (Morrison, Ellis, Morrison, Bearden, & Harriman, 2007). Adolescents may want their bodies to appear differently. While some things are outside of one's control without surgery (e.g., having a larger penis or breasts), there are times when adolescents can control their appearance (e.g., body mass index). While some comparisons certainly can be considered unhealthy, it should be noted that not all upward comparisons are dangerous.

Individuals who are more satisfied with the appearance of their sex-related body parts generally display a greater sexual confidence (Cranney, 2015). Young males tend to place more emphasis on the appearance of their genitals than do young females. The research has consistently found that there are no significant relationships between female's consumption of SEIM and genital self-image; however, the opposite has been found for young males (Cranney, 2015; Goldsmith, Dunkley, Dang, & Gorzalka, 2017). Perhaps this is because adolescent males place an extremely high importance on penis size, and young males may boast about having a larger-than-average penis. For many men, penis size represents masculinity and may be considered a requirement for satisfying a sexual partner. Young males who make comparisons in penis size to male Internet actors should proceed with caution as those comparisons may be flawed.

For many adolescents, both heterosexual and gay, physical appearance is of the utmost importance and comes under great social pressure. As much as SEIM depicts fantasy, it equally has the potential to depict reality. In actuality, the beauty of the individual body is still completely subjective. Contrary to what some believe, not all young people are interested in having the bodies or other physical characteristics resembling actors and actresses found in Internet pornography. For many adolescents who consume SEIM, the search is not for the ideal body or to achieve the attractiveness of a professional actor or actress. Some young males and women may prefer amateur pornography, which depicts other individuals who might be considered of average attractiveness because it is more realistic (Hald & Stulhofer, 2016). This is especially true for young people who may not consider themselves as attractive as their peers.

Young females tend to put greater emphasis on being as sexually desirable as their partners but are also at a higher risk of being sexually objectified (Janssen, Carpenter, & Graham, 2003). When we consider the idea of objectification, young people can either engage in the sexual objectification of others, accept an unhealthy objectification of themselves, or both. Although the effects of sexual objectification may not be immediate during adolescence, there is a significant possibility that such objectifications may present as mental health concerns later in adult life.

Body image

Body image is subjective and refers to how an individual thinks and feels about his or her physical appearance. For example, body type, shape, size, and physical attractiveness are all subjective evaluations that people can place on themselves. The way one conceptualizes body image is a significant contributor to one's overall identity as a human being and has the potential to either positively or negatively impact a client's psychological health. For example, a positive impact for individuals who are more satisfied with their own body image could be increased confidence in their own overall sexuality. This overall confidence with individual sexuality can result in greater sexual satisfaction and increased sexual self-esteem (Vogels, 2019). A negative body image may lead to a lack of sexual confidence and, ultimately, result in sexual avoidance (Goldsmith et al., 2017). An overall dissatisfaction with one's own body image significantly increases the chances that one could experience body dysmorphia (Cranney, 2015) and depression and experiment with unhealthy diets, unsafe exercise regimes, or expensive body-altering surgeries (Vogels, 2019).

Many individuals can be placed into categories based on one of three basic body types: *ectomorphic*, *mesomorphic*, and *endomorphic*. Ectomorphic individuals can be identified by a small frame size, a very low body fat ratio, and limited muscle mass (Merriam-Webster.com, n.d.). In other words, ectomorphs are generally considered to be thin but not necessarily unhealthy or underweight. On the opposite end of the body type spectrum are the endomorphs. Endomorphic individuals will present a much larger frame, a higher body fat ratio, and not much lean muscle (Merriam-Webster.com, n.d.). Individuals with this body type may appear to be thicker than average but are not necessarily unhealthy or overweight. Lastly, individuals carrying more of a medium frame with a lower body fat ratio and a higher muscle mass index are considered to have a mesomorphic body type (Law & Labre, 2002). Mesomorphs are generally considered to have the ideal body type and are likely viewed by others as having an ideal form (Law & Labre, 2002), being both strong and healthy. Individuals with mesomorphic body types are found extensively in marketing campaigns that use perceived physical attractiveness to market products and make those products more appealing. Because this body type is considered appealing to so many, mesomorphs are very commonly found in Internet pornography.

Both heterosexual and homosexual consumers of SEIM are more likely to find young, athletic, muscular, and physically attractive actors and actresses, which tends to be consistent with body ideals. However, the bodies of professional actors and actresses depicted in Internet pornography are not always representative of the general consumer population (Goldsmith et al., 2017; Millward, 2013; Peter & Valkenburg, 2014). In fact, the body types depicted in SEIM are often impossible for most adolescents to obtain without dangerous behaviors and surgical procedures (Vogels, 2019). Female pornography actresses tend to be curvaceously thin with an average to large bust, a smaller waist, and rounder hips. The average female professional pornography actress weighs roughly 117 pounds and displays measurements of a 34-inch bust, 24-inch waist, and 34-inch hips (Millward, 2013). In comparison, the average American female weighs nearly 45 pounds more with roughly a 12-inch-larger waist (Vogels, 2019). Male actors tend to carry a low amount of body fat and appear to have a more muscular lean build. The average male professional pornography actor weighs nearly 168 pounds (Millward, 2013), which is roughly 19 pounds heavier than the average American male (Vogels, 2019).

When adolescents consume SEIM, they are constantly exposed to the ideal mesomorphic body, which teaches them about how they should look and what their body types should be (Tylka, 2015). However, when Internet pornography becomes the frame of reference, it is possible that expectations about one's appearance may become distorted or unrealistic. For example, female pornography actresses exhibit body images that are mostly unrealistic and unobtainable; however, many young females will notice that pornography actresses typically represent a body type that is commonly accepted as ideal. When internalized, a young female may begin to develop insecurities about her own body image (Löfgren-Mårtenson & Månsson, 2010), which can lead to other sexual concerns. For example, research has shown that when women believe they should physically resemble the actresses they see in SEIM, they are more susceptible to experiencing sexual dissatisfaction (Stewart & Szymanski, 2012). It is important for young females to recognize the unrealistic ideal body type portrayed in Internet pornography and having such self-awareness may deter against experiencing dissatisfaction with body image.

Similar to their female counterparts, young males who compare their own bodies to the ideal mesomorphic body types portrayed in Internet pornography may also experience body dissatisfaction (Elder, Brooks, & Morrow, 2012; Vogels, 2019). Some adolescent males may compromise their physical health in order to obtain the body type they see in SEIM as ideal and attractive to their sexual partners (Tylka, 2015). In order to obtain this physical appearance, some adolescent males may engage in dangerous dieting or exercise regimens, and this may lead to unsafe uses of anabolic steroids or surgical body altering procedures (Tylka, 2015).

Male members of the LGBTQ community typically experience greater body dissatisfaction than heterosexual males (Martins, Tiggemann, & Kirkbride, 2007), and taking the risk to physically alter one's body in an unhealthy way is significantly greater for gay and bisexual males who experience body dissatisfaction (Hadland, Austin, Goodenow, & Calzo, 2014). Body dissatisfaction in the LGBTQ community may also have a significant impact on one's self-esteem. When gay and bisexual males have a body type that is closer to what is considered ideal in the LGBTQ community, these males report higher levels of self-esteem than those who have other body types that are assumed to be less than ideal (Kvalem, Træen, & Iantaffi, 2016).

Interestingly, one does not even need to consume Internet pornography to experience its potential impact on body image. For example, it is not uncommon for women to question if their male partners are comparing their bodies to the bodies of actresses in Internet pornography. Many young females may begin to question their own sexual desirability when they believe their partners are comparing their bodies to the assumed ideal type found in SEIM (Tylka & Kroon Van Diest, 2015). This comparison may lead to conflicts, sexual dissatisfaction, and other relational concerns.

As helpers who work with adolescents, the importance of body image cannot be stressed enough. How we work with young people as they develop opinions about their own bodies can be critical as they develop physically, sexually, and emotionally. We invite readers to consider the questions posed in Learning Activity 5.1 and how those reflections can be used as they think about working with adolescents and their consumption of SEIM.

Learning Activity 5.1

Reflections on our own self-image

Consider the following questions and their relationship to adolescents and SEIM. Specifically, the first three questions ask you to think about adolescents and their use of SEIM. Questions 4–6 challenge you to reflect on your own experiences and how you may draw from those experiences in your practice.

Questions for thought and discussion:
1. How might an individual's body image be positively or negatively impacted by the consumption of Internet pornography?
2. Having an understanding of how body image could directly influence individual sexuality, what other factors related to Internet pornography consumption might impact youth self-esteem?
3. What other social comparisons can be made by sexually developing youth who may consume Internet pornography?

Questions for further reflection:
4. Consider your own body type now and how it differs from your child and adolescent years. How has your body satisfaction changed over time?
5. Are there any factors that may have driven a desire to modify your own body? Is a healthy body more important that an attractive one?
6. What role does your own body image play in your sexuality? What impact does body image and individual sexual confidence have on your own self-esteem?

Physical attractiveness

The idea of physical attractiveness is subjective, or as the idiom goes, "beauty is in the eye of the beholder." Most people have preferences for what they find attractive in a sexual partner, and most people select sexual partners with similar levels of physical attractiveness (Shaw, Taylor, Fiore, Mendelsohn, & Cheshire, 2011). For example, if we consider attractiveness on a scale of 1 to 10, where 1 is considered not at all attractive and 10 very attractive, a given adolescent may rate him or herself a 5, or average. The consumption of SEIM may prove an opportunity for that person to fantasize about having a sexual encounter with someone who is physically much more attractive than they believe themselves to be, perhaps someone they would rate as an 8 or 9 on the 10-point scale. However, what we find is that people are, in realty, physically attracted to others whom they find equally attractive as themselves. Consider again the example of someone who rates him or herself a 5 out of 10. That person is more likely to be attracted to someone he or she considers somewhere between a 4 and a 6 than someone who rates a 9 or 10.

The fantasy sought after in SEIM is not always having a sexual relationship with a significantly more attractive partner but may be with a partner who one considers more realistic. Individuals seeking out a more realistic fantasy online may be less drawn to professionally and digitally altered Internet pornography but instead gravitate toward SEIM that features amateur actors and actresses or Internet pornography that is homemade. Many adolescents prefer amateur Internet pornography over that which is professionally produced (Vogels, 2019).

In the end, individuals may compare themselves or their partners' body types and physical attractiveness to the actors and actresses depicted in Internet pornography. However, it is important for helping professionals to understand that these types of comparisons are not necessarily negative and can sometimes be positive for adolescent sexual development. For example, professional pornography actors and actresses may appear to be good role models for body positivity (Vogels, 2019), and many youth may be inspired by these aesthetic ideals and strive to achieve similar attributes in a healthy way. Another potential positive outcome of consuming SEIM is that adolescents may be exposed to a wide variety of body types and may have the opportunity to expand their definitions of physical beauty. Increasing one's knowledge of the variability of body types can lead to acceptance of one's own appearance (Kvalem et al., 2016). Finally, regarding the proliferation of amateur actors and actresses and homemade Internet pornography, it is possible that adolescents who seek out more realistic body types may develop more realistic body type standards themselves (Vogels, 2019).

Genitalia and other sexual-related body parts

Some adolescents will experience concerns over the appearance and functioning of their genitalia and other sexual body parts (e.g., penis, vagina, breasts); these concerns can impact their opinions of their overall self-image. When we consider adolescent consumption of SEIM, it is important to attend to the fact that sexualized body parts are continuously on display and are usually the focus of the sexual acts depicted in Internet pornography (Goldsmith et al., 2017). The focus on specific body parts in SEIM may lead adolescents to take note of the differences between their own bodies and those that are depicted in much of what is available online. For example, while adolescence is a time of physical development, which usually results in the growth of pubic hair, many of the actors and actresses found in SEIM do not display public hair (Morrison et al., 2007).

Female actresses in Internet pornography appear to display a smaller or tighter labia majora (outer folds of skin) and labia minora (inner folds of skin), which enclose the genitals. However, research findings suggest that there are no significant associations between female consumption of Internet pornography and perception of one's genitals (Vogels, 2019). Female actresses in Internet pornography also usually display breasts that are average to above average in size. Although the size and shapes of breasts are a common focus of SEIM, female consumers are generally not concerned with breast size (Cranney, 2015; Vogels, 2019). One explanation for this is that many adolescents may already possess this body characteristic and, therefore, not find it concerning. Another explanation is that adolescent girls are not necessarily attending to the breast size of women depicted in SEIM. Young females are constantly exposed to other female's breasts, both in sexualized media but also in everyday life, while young males are not often exposed to other men's erect penises (Cranney, 2015). As a result, young females may not place the same amount of concern on the size of their breasts as a male would on the size of his penis.

Regarding relationships between SEIM consumption and satisfaction with the size of one's penis, research findings are mixed (Cranney, 2015; Peter & Valkenburg, 2014); however, some have suggested that the onset of such concerns may relate directly to consumption of SEIM during youth (Ghanem et al., 2007; Shamloul, 2005). It may be difficult to draw a conclusion that adolescent consumption of SEIM leads directly to concerns about the size of one's penis. However, the research suggests that these factors may be correlated. In cases where Internet pornography is used as a frame of reference for penis size standards, young consumers will almost always have a recognizably smaller penis than the pornography actor. If an adolescent male internalizes these thoughts, then a negative self-image may be the result, and an adolescent male may develop a belief that he is sexually inadequate (Veale et al., 2014). For example, young males could become self-conscious about sexual situations or even embarrassed to be seen naked.

In conclusion, consuming Internet pornography has the potential to both positively and negatively impact adolescent self-image. For adolescent girls, they may compare their breasts or vaginal areas with those of the actresses found in SEIM; however, the belief that certain characteristics are preferred (e.g., firm breasts or smaller vaginal features) may be mitigated by the fact that these characteristics are often found in younger women naturally. The negative impacts of breast size or genital self-image on women may not come until later in life. For young males, genital self-image is more likely to be experienced earlier during youth. For some, concerns about penis size could last only during adolescence, but could also be a concern throughout life.

Individuals who are more satisfied with the appearance of their sex-related body parts generally display a greater sexual satisfaction (Cranney, 2015).

For many individuals, regardless of age, sexual interactions can produce a significant amount of anxiety when such high standards are being placed upon an ideal body image. Individuals may experience sexual dissatisfaction when a preoccupation with body image becomes a cognitive distraction (Goldsmith et al., 2017). For example, it may be extremely difficult for an individual to fully engage in a romantic and intimate sexual relationship if concerned with his or her body image or other underlying issues related to self-confidence.

Self-esteem

Given the various issues discussed in this chapter, it is certainly possible that consumption of SEIM can negatively impact the self-esteem of the adolescents who consume it. For example, young consumers of Internet pornography may develop attitudes about gender roles and sexual behavior that are both unrealistic and unhealthy (see Chapter 3 for more on issues related to attitudes and beliefs). The stereotypical male gender role portrays the actor in Internet pornography as dominant, superior, and in a position of power. Inaccurate portrayals of masculinity and genders roles in Internet pornography can potentially be internalized by young people (McCreary, Saucier, & Courtenay, 2005) or even be projected by adolescents onto sexual partners or others.

A significant amount of Internet pornography displays women responding positively to sexual objectification by men; however, this objectification is seldom welcome in the real world outside of the Internet. In reality, young females who accept this sexual objectification as the norm incorrectly learn that sexual partners should be submissive, inferior, and powerless. Sexually objectified females may find themselves expected to engage in sexual acts or behaviors that they find to be uncomfortable or undesirable (Bergner & Bridges, 2002), which may ultimately challenge adolescent women to question their self-worth (Tylka & Kroon Van Diest, 2015). It is possible that some women who were sexually objectified in adolescence may experience greater relationship anxiety, ultimately impacting their adult romantic relationships Tylka & Kroon Van Diest, 2015). Additionally, women who were sexually objectified are at an increased risk of developing lower self-esteem, which may present itself during youth or later in adulthood (Tylka & Kroon Van Diest, 2015). In theory, sexual objectification may lead the objectified individual to self-objectify or adopt a partner's sexual perception (Tylka & Kroon Van Diest, 2015). People who view themselves as submissive, inferior, and powerless sexual objects may begin to accept and conform to that unhealthy role expectation.

Vogels (2019) found positive associations with the consumption of sexually explicit material. A positive factor associated with consuming Internet pornography is the possibility to empower individuals to think, act, and behave in a more sexually confident way (Vogels, 2019). For example, her study suggests that males and females alike could gain higher self-esteem through exposure to sexually explicit material. In addition, Vogels (2019) also suggests the possibility of an increased body satisfaction for males and a greater comfort level being naked for females. It is possible that this increased sexual confidence may encourage some to stop projecting sexual encounters online and start pursuing healthy romantic relationships in reality.

Conclusion

In conclusion, society defines body ideals, which are disseminated through various types of media. In a culture that includes SEIM, where the naked body is on display and a much greater emphasis is placed on the sexual-related body parts, body ideals have the potential to become greatly distorted to adolescents who are experiencing significant physical and emotional development. As technology continues to advance and evolve, Internet pornography can easily be digitally altered to more closely conform to the notions of an ideal body. When internalized, Internet pornography consumption has the potential to impact how young individuals view body ideals, which can lead to their own body dissatisfaction.

Helping professionals working with adolescent males and females who consume SEIM will need to explore potential internalized beliefs related to body image, genital self-image, and the impact that self-image has on self-esteem. While these conversations may be difficult, as helpers, we have a responsibility to educate young males and females on these issues. If we do not attend to the role SEIM can play in the development of self-image, we are doing a disservice to our clients. Learning Activity 5.2 provides a case illustration depicting how helpers may be challenged to work with adolescent clients around these issues.

Learning Activity 5.2

The case of Jenny and Bryan

Jenny is a client of yours in your therapeutic practice. Jenny and her boyfriend, Bryan, are 16-year-old high school students who have been dating for the last several months. Like many adolescent youth, both are in the midst of their sexual development and have recently become physically intimate with one another. For both adolescents, this is the first introduction to sexual intercourse. Like many young males, Bryan has had some exposure to what to expect during intercourse through his use of Internet pornography. However, his partner, Jenny, has never had any exposure to Internet pornography . . . until now.

Although Jenny and Bryan have only had intercourse on a few occasions, both have admitted that being sexually intimate was not exactly what they each expected. Taking some advice from a friend to help improve their sexual relationship, Bryan suggested to Jenny that she watch pornography with him on the Internet. Jenny believes she will be in a relationship with Bryan for the rest of her life, and she is more than willing to do anything that will make Bryan happy. Like many adolescent couples, Jenny is now watching Internet pornography with Bryan.

While watching Internet pornography together, Jenny has made some observations, which, ultimately, have led her to compare herself, and her partner, to what she has seen online. Jenny sees Bryan as thinner and less muscular than the actors in the pornography they have viewed, and he has a smaller penis. She has never thought about this before, but she is beginning to wonder if penis size is related to good sex because she does not get much sexual pleasure from her lovemaking with Bryan. Jenny also noticed that the men in the videos seem to be able to engage in sex forever. Bryan tends to only last a few minutes during sex, which she is now wondering about. Is that normal?

But, overall, probably the most surprising observation to Jenny is the way Internet pornography actresses look, behave, and seem to enjoy sex. Jenny has observed that the actresses tend to be much thinner and have much larger breasts than she does. Not only does Jenny begin to question whether her physical appearance is abnormal but also wonders what brings a female to sexual ecstasy so quickly and easily.

Jenny has always believed she was carrying a little extra weight and that her breasts were small, but now she has become completely uncomfortable being naked in front of Bryan. Jenny has since convinced herself that Bryan is only interested in girls with the body types similar to those of the actresses they see online. During intercourse with Bryan, all Jenny can think about is what Bryan is thinking. Does he wonder why she doesn't look like the actresses in the videos? He gets aroused when he watches them, so is that what he wants or expects?

Jenny has placed a great amount of importance on physical desirability to Bryan; she is currently considering a number of options about how she can change her body to better please him. Some options are extremely unhealthy. She has cut back her caloric intake and is exercising constantly. She has considered having cosmetic surgery to increase the size of her breasts, but her parents have refused to agree to the procedure. "That's fine," she says angrily. "I'll wait until I'm 18, and I'll save the money up myself."

To make matters worse, Jenny is also concerned that something is wrong with her sexual functioning as she does not seem to be enjoying sexual intercourse with Bryan as much as the actresses do in Internet pornography.

What are the most serious issues as you consider Jenny's case? How might you address these concerns with her? What are the challenges you anticipate in your work with Jenny?

Summary

- For adolescents who are still developing sexually, the inaccurate portrayal of sexuality found in SEIM significantly increases the risk of internalizing such unrealistic expectations. An unhealthy internalization of unrealistic sexual expectations can encourage developing youth to hold themselves to very high and unattainable standards.

- Through a process of social comparison, many people internalize body image based on the appearance of other individuals. People with greater satisfaction about their bodies tend to display greater sexual confidence.
- For many youth, both heterosexual and gay, physical appearance is of the utmost importance and comes under great social pressure.
- The way an individual conceptualizes body image is a significant contributor to one's overall identity as a human being and, as such, has the potential to either positively or negatively impact a client's psychological health.
- Many individuals can be placed into categories based on one of three basic body types: *ectomorphic*, *mesomorphic*, and *endomorphic*.
- When adolescents consume SEIM, they may take cues from these media about how they should look, what their body types should be, and assume that what they see in these images and videos is the ideal. However, when Internet pornography becomes the frame of reference, it is possible that expectations about one's appearance may become distorted or unrealistic.
- Most people have preferences for what they find attractive in a sexual partner, and most people consider their own physical attractiveness when engaging in sexual fantasy about what they find attractive in others.
- Concerns over genitalia and other sexual body parts can impact the development of self-image in adolescents. These body parts are on constant display and are the focus of much SEIM. These concerns can impact both young males and women.
- A significant amount of Internet pornography may show females positively responding to being sexually objectified by males; however, this objectification is seldom welcome in the real world outside of the Internet. If these portrayals of women are internalized, healthy development of self-esteem can be impacted in adolescent girls.

Additional resources

In print

Löfgren-Mårtenson, L., & Månsson, S. (2010). Lust, love, and life: A qualitative study of Swedish adolescents' perceptions and experiences with pornography. *Journal of Sex Research, 47*, 568–579. doi:10.1080/00224490903151374

Peter, J., & Valkenburg, P. M. (2014). Does exposure to sexually explicit Internet material increase body dissatisfaction? A longitudinal study. *Computers in Human Behavior, 36*, 297–307. doi:10.1016/j.chb.2014.03.071

On the web

Millward, J. (2013, February). *Deep inside: A study of 10,000 porn stars and their careers.* Retrieved from http://jonmillward.com/blog/studies/deep-inside-a-study-of-10000-porn-stars/

References

Bergner, R. M., & Bridges, A. J. (2002). The significance of heavy pornography involvement for romantic partners: Research and clinical implications. *Journal of Sex & Marital Therapy, 28*, 193–206. doi:10.1080/009262302760328235

Cranney, S. (2015). Internet pornography use and sexual body image in a Dutch sample. *International Journal of Sexual Health*, *27*(3), 316–323. doi:10.1080/19317611.2014.9 99967

Ectomorphic. (n.d.). *In Merriam-Webster.com*. Retrieved from www.merriam-webster.com/dictionary/ectomorphic

Elder, W. B., Brooks, G. R., & Morrow, S. L. (2012). Sexual self-schemas of heterosexual men. *Psychology of Men & Masculinity*, *13*, 166–179. doi:10.1037/a0024835

Endomorphic. (n.d.). *In Merriam-Webster.com*. Retrieved from www.merriam-webster.com/dictionary/endomorphic

Ghanem, H., Shamloul, R., Khodeir, F., ElShafie, H., Kaddah, A., & Ismail, I. (2007). Structured management and counseling for patients with a complaint of a small penis. *The Journal of Sexual Medicine*, *4*, 1322–1327. doi:10.1111/j.1743-6109.2007.00463.x

Goldsmith, K., Dunkley, C. R., Dang, S. S., & Gorzalka, B. B. (2017). Pornography consumption and its association with sexual concerns and expectations among young males and women. *The Canadian Journal of Human Sexuality*, *26*(2), 151–162. doi:10.3138/cjhs.262-a2

Hadland, S. E., Austin, S. B., Goodenow, C. S., & Calzo, J. P. (2014). Weight misperception and unhealthy weight control behaviors among sexual minorities in the general adolescent population. *Journal of Adolescent Health*, *54*, 296–303. doi:10.1016/j.jadohealth.2013.08.021

Hald, G. M., & Stulhofer, A. (2016). What types of pornography do people use and do they cluster? Assessing types and categories of pornography consumption in a large-scale online sample. *Journal of Sex Research*, *53*(7), 849–859. doi:10.1080/00224499.2015.1 065953

Janssen, E., Carpenter, D., & Graham, C. A. (2003). Selecting films for sex research: Gender differences in erotic film preference. *Archives of Sexual Behavior*, *32*, 243–251. doi:10.1023/A:1023413617648

Kvalem, I. L., Træen, B., & Iantaffi, A. (2016). Internet pornography use, body ideals, and sexual self-esteem in Norwegian gay and bisexual men. *Journal of Homosexuality*, *63*(4), 522–540. doi:10.1080/00918369.2015.1083782

Law, C., & Labre, M. P. (2002). Cultural standards of attractiveness: A thirty-year look at changes in male images in magazines. *Journalism & Mass Communication Quarterly*, *79*(3), 697–711. doi:10.1177/107769900207900310

Löfgren-Mårtenson, L., & Månsson, S. (2010). Lust, love, and life: A qualitative study of Swedish adolescents' perceptions and experiences with pornography. *Journal of Sex Research*, *47*, 568–579. doi:10.1080/00224490903151374

Martins, Y., Tiggemann, M., & Kirkbride, A. (2007). Those Speedos become them: The role of self-objectification in gay and heterosexual men's body image. *Personality and Social Psychology Bulletin*, *33*, 634–647. doi:10.1177/0146167206297403

McCreary, D. R., Saucier, D. M., & Courtenay, W. H. (2005). The drive for muscularity and masculinity: Testing the associations among gender role traits, behaviors, attitudes, and conflict. *Psychology of Men and Masculinity*, *6*, 83–94. doi:10.1037/1524-9220.6.2.83

Millward, J. (2013, February). *Deep inside: A study of 10,000 porn stars and their careers*. Retrieved from http://jonmillward.com/blog/studies/deep-inside-a-study-of-10000-porn-stars/

Morrison, T. G., Ellis, S. R., Morrison, M. A., Bearden, A., & Harriman, R. L. (2007). Exposure to sexually explicit material and variations in body esteem, genital attitudes, and sexual esteem among a sample of Canadian Men. *The Journal of Men's Studies*, *14*(2), 209–222. doi:10.3149/jms.1402.209

Peter, J., & Valkenburg, P. M. (2014). Does exposure to sexually explicit Internet material increase body dissatisfaction? A longitudinal study. *Computers in Human Behavior, 36*, 297–307. doi:10.1016/j.chb.2014.03.071

Self-Esteem [Def. 1]. (n.d.). *Merriam-Webster Online*. In Merriam-Webster. Retrieved from www.merriam-webster.com/dictionary/self-esteem

Shamloul, R. (2005). Treatment of men complaining of short penis. *Urology, 65*(6), 1183–1185. doi:10.1016/j.urology.2004.12.066

Shaw Taylor, L., Fiore, A. T., Mendelsohn, G. A., & Cheshire, C. (2011). "Out of my league": A real-world test of the matching hypothesis. *Personality and Social Psychology Bulletin, 37*(7), 942–954. doi:10.1177/0146167211409947

Stewart, D. N., & Szymanski, D. M. (2012). Young adult female's reports of their male romantic partner's pornography use as a correlate of their self-esteem, relationship quality, and sexual satisfaction. *Sex Roles, 67*, 257–271. doi:10.1007/s11199-012-0164-0

Tylka, T. L. (2015). No harm in looking, right? Men's pornography consumption, body image, and well-being. *Psychology of Men & Masculinity, 16*(1), 97–107. doi:10.1037/a0035774

Tylka, T. L., & Kroon Van Diest, A. M. (2015). You looking at her "hot" body may not be "cool" for me: Integrating male partners' pornography use into objectification theory for women. *Psychology of Women Quarterly, 39*(1), 67–84. doi:10.1177/0361684314521784

Veale, D., Eshkevari, E., Read, J., Miles, S., Troglia, A., Phillips, R., . . . Muir, G. (2014). Beliefs about penis size. *Journal of Sexual Medicine, 11*, 84–92. doi:10.1111/jsm.12294

Vogels, E. A. (2019). Loving oneself: The associations among sexually explicit media, body image, and perceived realism. *The Journal of Sex Research, 56*(6), 778–790. doi:10.1080/00224499.2018.1475546

6 From the self to the world
The intersection of pornography and culture

The Ryans are a traditional conservative Irish Catholic family. On any typical night in the Ryan household, the father would arrive home from his second job, and mom would prepare a family dinner. The children in the family looked forward to family dinners as well, each taking a turn in leading the family in prayer. After dinner, the family would typically watch the evening news together. One of the rules in the Ryan household was that dad controlled what his children watched on television, and he never deviated from his favorite conservative cable news channel.

The top news story this particular evening covered breaking news of accusations that a local politician was caught having an affair with an adult film actress. The news reported that this would be the political scandal of the century, as the adult film actress had accepted campaign finances for her silence about the affair. Repeatedly, the news reporter used the term "porn star" in his description of the politician's mistress. Without hesitation, dad changed from one channel to another, which never happened before. What dad found on every news channel that evening was the breaking news about an adult film actress having an affair with a high-ranking politician. The topic of sex was something on which dad held very strict religious views, and the idea of pornography was considered disgusting and appalling.

Intrigued by his father's unique behavior, Matthew Ryan asked, "Why can't we watch the story about the porn star?" Dad replied, "We don't talk about that filth in this house and that's fake news! Now go to your room!"

Upset by his father's outburst, Matthew ran to his room as his father ordered. Wanting to know more, Matthew did what he has done every time he's wanted to learning something for school: he opened his laptop. Matthew typed the words "porn star" into his unfiltered Internet search engine and clicked enter. To his surprise, what seemed to be a million sexually explicit videos were now available to view, free of charge. Over the course of the next several weeks, Matthew would retreat to his room where he would continue to view hundreds of pornographic videos on the Internet.

Matthew knew that his mother and father would never approve of his discovery, so he hid his laptop as best he could. But one day, Matthew was running late for school and left his laptop open on his nightstand and ran off to class. While mom was cleaning the house that afternoon, she came across Matthew's laptop with pornography visible on the screen. Mom immediately called dad home from work that day because she could not put into words over the phone what she viewed. Both mom and dad awaited Matthew's arrival home from school, but neither of them was comfortable enough to discuss with Matthew what he has been watching online. Instead, Matthew was driven directly to St. Vincent's Parish where he would spend the next month in intensive "counseling" with Father Mike, who promised to save Matthew from his sinful behavior.

As the Internet has expanded throughout a sexualized society and a multicultural world, the pornography industry has become farther reaching than ever before. As adolescents grow within a digital age, their exposure to various types of SEIM will continue to increase. For many youth, Internet pornography will be their first introduction to sexuality and culture will be a significant factor of when and why this introduction will take place. Some adolescents will intentionally consume Internet pornography as a means to satisfy a curiosity, strengthen a sexual knowledge, or fulfill a sexual desire. Others will find that the consumption of Internet pornography was accidental. Regardless of the reason for consuming SEIM, helping professionals will find that adolescents' understanding of sexuality is nontraditional; their sexual education in areas such as reproductive functioning and sexual health exists in a world of diverse sexuality. Different cultural perspectives exist in relation to SEIM; the purpose of this chapter is to give the reader a multicultural overview from a neutral perspective. This perspective exists where Internet pornography intersects with age, gender, worldview, sexual identity, political ideology, and religion.

Regardless of how youth are introduced to SEIM, it is imperative that helping professionals recognize the importance of culture, or as the American Counseling Association (ACA) states in the *2014 Code of Ethics*, counselors "recognize that culture affects the manner in which clients' problems are defined and experienced" (American Counseling Association, 2014, Standard E.5.b.). This chapter will examine how cultural factors, such as age, gender, political ideology, worldview, religion, and sexual identity influence youth consumption of Internet pornography. After reading this chapter, you should be able to

1 Understand the impact of age on Internet pornography consumption;
2 Understand gender from a biological, psychological, and social perspective and how such perspectives can influence adolescent consumption of SEIM;
3 Recognize that political ideology influences the consumption of Internet pornography;
4 Be cognizant of how worldviews may influence SEIM consumption;
5 Understand the theologically based sexual values of religious youth and the potential for cognitive dissonance that can result from viewing SEIM; and
6 Develop an awareness of Internet pornography consumption from the perspective of sexual identity.

Age

Human sexuality is present in the development of individuals from birth through adulthood and is a natural and essential part of the overall personal, social, and emotional development of all youth (Behun, Cerrito, Delmonico, & Campenni,

2017). As the Internet continues to grow and evolve, the availability of pornography will continue to increase around the world. For many adolescents with online access, an increase in the availability of SEIM will likely make both the intentional and unintentional consumption of Internet pornography nearly unavoidable (see Chapter 1 for more on intentional and unintentional SEIM consumption). Therefore, one should assume that children can unintentionally consume pornography as early as their fine motor skills allow them to maneuver electronic devices with Internet access. We can expect that nearly all male, and roughly two-thirds of female, youth will be exposed to pornography online prior to reaching adulthood.

For adolescents, exposure to pornography is expected to increase with age, considering the sexual development from childhood through adolescence, the hormonal impact of puberty, and the peer pressure to understand sexuality (Rasmussen & Bierman, 2016). Older youth will likely be more deliberate in their consumption of Internet pornography and more likely to experience enjoyment of SEIM than their younger peers. Conversely, younger viewers are less interested in Internet pornography than their older peers because they have not yet matured to a place where they have interest in sexuality (Tsaliki, 2011). This lack of sexual maturity will make younger online users more likely to consume Internet pornography accidentally and increases the likelihood that these youth may find the experience to be disgusting or offensive.

In contrast, a significant majority of youth do not necessarily agree that pornography is harmful when it adheres to culturally acceptable norms (Tsaliki, 2011), and many adolescents consider the consumption of pornography to be a healthy and normal expression of sexuality (Hald & Malamuth, 2008). While young people may not believe that SEIM is harmful, the negative outcomes that could result from consuming SIEM may not be immediately apparent. (Willoughby, Carroll, Nelson, & Padilla-Walker, 2014). Helping professionals working with youth should be cautioned that not all exposure to pornography will result in negative effects.

Gender

Generally speaking, adolescents are at a particularly vulnerable time in their sexual development. Although most mainstream research describes gender as being either male or female, or the sex assigned at birth, not all youth will identify with their assigned gender. It is important for the helping professional to understand that gender extends beyond anatomical or biological aspects of being male or female and youth should be respected by the gender with which they most identify. Male, female, and gender-neutral youth may have different reasons for seeking out Internet pornography.

Considering youth gender differences in SEIM consumption from a social perspective, it is not uncommon for many young males to watch pornography together for reasons other than education or sexual arousal. It is also not uncommon for young males to be pressured into watching pornography. For many young men, viewing SEIM may be considered a rite of passage in terms of sexual development (Beggan & Allison, 2003).

When we examine consumption of SEIM from a more scientific perspective, adolescent males report seeking sexual content from SEIM at significantly higher rates than females (Bleakley, Hennessy, & Fishbein, 2011), and the consumption of pornography for young males tends to increase over time (Ma & Shek, 2013). It is possible that the increase in testosterone in adolescent males may be a contributing factor in the likelihood that one will engage in SEIM consumption (Baumeister, 2000). It is also possible that the greater prevalence of masturbation among young males may be a contributing factor to the finding that young males tend to view SEIM more frequently than their female peers (Træen, Nilsen, & Stigum, 2006).

For adolescent females, the consumption of pornography is shown to have increased over the past few decades (Lykke & Cohen, 2015), and females are believed to consume pornography at a greater frequency than their contemporaries did in previous generations (Diamond, 2009). Two explanations for this increase in SEIM consumption by young females include changing gender dynamics and a greater willingness among young females to engage in sexual exploration (Cooper & Klein, 2017). Another reason for the uptick in female SEIM consumption might be related to with whom pornography is consumed. Female pornography consumption has consistently been connected to their partners' use, and heterosexual females are more likely to view Internet pornography with their partners than they are to view it alone (Træen et al., 2006). In theory, as male Internet pornography consumption increases, female consumption should increase as well.

Political ideology

For many, Internet pornography consumption is closely related to political ideologies, and those philosophies may include strong, personally sensitive values. Pornography has been the topic of public policy and controversy for many decades, and with advancements in technology, pornography will continue to be present in public debate for many decades to come (see the chapter on current issues in this text for more on these topics). At the center of many philosophical debates surrounding pornography, one will find both far-left liberal and far-right conservative arguments pitting individual liberty against societal morality. However, there is some common ground. One common belief held worldwide is that children and adolescents are a vulnerable population in need of greater protections from potential causes of harm. As the age of the consumer of SEIM decreases, the potential harm that may be experienced by the consumer increases. For example, children are more likely going to have much more negative reaction to SEIM than adolescents who are approaching adulthood. At the cultural intersection of sexual ideology, there will always remain a positive and negative stance that considers the impacts of Internet pornography on youth.

Adolescents who hold more liberal or positive attitudes toward sexuality are more likely to be frequent consumers of SEIM. Those who hold more liberal beliefs related to pornography indicate a tendency to believe that it is an individual's right to choose to produce, consume, or participate in pornography within the stipulations of the law (Häggström-Nordin, Sandberg, Hanson, & Tydén, 2006).

Regarding the law, while liberal ideologies tend to take a more relaxed perspective on SEIM, child pornography is almost never considered acceptable. Those who hold liberal beliefs are more likely to view sex as a recreational activity that can be intended for purposes of pleasure. Individuals considered to be slightly liberal to extremely liberal are more likely consumers of SEIM than their conservative peers and tend to share a more positive opinion on diverse sexual practices and hold stronger stances on LGBTQ rights to equal marriage (Frutos & Merrill, 2017).

Contrary to the liberal belief that the viewing of pornography is an individual's right, a more conservative philosophy would protect the individual from the potential harm pornography can inflict. Many conservatives believe that love and sexuality are not independent of one another and that sexuality is meant to be something shared only between a married couple (Häggström-Nordin et al., 2006). Additionally, conservative-minded individuals are more likely to view sexuality as an activity that is solely for the purpose of procreation. Therefore, for many conservatives, the consumption of pornography carries a negative connotation and is considered an issue of immorality. Not surprisingly, individuals who consider themselves slightly conservative to extremely conservative are likely to report lower consumption of Internet pornography (Frutos & Merrill, 2017).

In addition to general conservative and liberal perspectives, another consideration is the potential incongruence between a woman's right to express her sexuality contrasted with the concepts of sexual exploitation and manipulation. Although it is possible that some may see pornography as a liberating expression of equal sexuality for women, this perspective is not necessarily common. In other words, many feminists consider pornography to be degrading to females. Many feminist thinkers believe that pornography, which places males in a role of superiority, is an exploitation of female bodies for the purposes of economic gain and an unethical act that is harmful to females (Häggström-Nordin et al., 2006).

Worldview

The worldviews of children and adolescents must be considered when considering the intersection of SEIM and culture. For the purpose of this text, two major worldviews are considered based on the major customs and traditions which separate Western and non-Western regions. Western cultures, such as those found in the North and South America, Australia, and throughout Europe, tend to have more liberal sexual views. Non-Western cultures can be found in Africa, Asia, and throughout the Middle East and, as a collective culture, tend to hold more conservative sexual values. Perhaps the most significant difference between these two major regions comes down to the issue of morality. The likelihood of SEIM consumption will be higher in communities where pornography is not considered a key issue and not believed to impact the overall moral functioning of society (Perry & Schleifer, 2017).

In Western cultures, the consumption of SEIM is becoming increasingly culturally acceptable (Cooper & Klein, 2017). Many adolescents have never known a world without the Internet, as it has been accessible in both public and private arenas for several decades, resulting in an entire generation of digital natives (see Chapter 2 for a more detailed discussion of digital natives). Digital natives and Western youth have only ever known one primary method of accessing pornography, which has been online. For many Western cultures, the overwhelming popularity and accessibility of the Internet has been a dominant source for youth seeking to fulfill a sexual curiosity, gain a deeper sexual understanding, or satisfy a sexual desire. The consumption of Internet pornography is unsurprisingly more likely for youth in Western cultures when compared to their non-Western counterparts. Although lower levels of Internet pornography consumption are being observed in non-Western cultures, these levels of exposure will only increase as Internet access becomes more readily available around the world.

In many non-Western cultures, Internet pornography is widely labeled as a danger to youth sexual development and a detriment to society. In many Asian countries, for example, pornography is heavily censored, as some governments try to protect the public from the immoral and offensive behaviors they believe to be on display (Mohd Azizuddin, 2011). It is a common belief in non-Western countries that pornography does not contribute anything to society; rather, it negatively impacts many cultural values (Mohd Azizuddin, 2011). Therefore, adolescents in non-Western cultures receive less sexual education in school and receive fewer messages regarding sexuality in the media; they may, therefore, go online to seek out additional information about sexuality. Based on the rapid expansion of technology and online access in both Western and non-Western cultures, Internet pornography has the potential to become the most sought out source of sexual education for many youth across the world.

Religion

The consumption of Internet pornography and its intersection with religion are deeply rooted in a near century-long debate. Long before the creation of the Internet, religions around the world have been on the forefront of combating pornography from its production, to its dissemination, and ending with its consumption (Perry, 2018). Historically, some religious groups and religious people tend to hold more theologically conservative sexual values, share many concerns, and overwhelmingly have negative views on pornography and its consumption. Among many religions is a common belief that the act of pornography is itself immoral, sinful, and violates deeply held religious standards.

In comparison to those with no religious affiliation, those who identify with a religion are more likely to hold a significantly stronger belief that the consumption of pornography leads to a breakdown in morals (Patterson & Price, 2012). Individuals who identify as religious have been found to be less likely to consume Internet pornography (Rasmussen & Bierman, 2016). It may be that religion teaches people how to avoid media that contributes to a disruption of individual moral principles (Perry, 2018). However, it is important to note that regardless of religious affiliation, youth still show an increase in consumption of SEIM as they get older (Rasmussen & Bierman, 2016).

Researchers have offered many explanations for the relationships found between religious practice and pornography consumption, although the directions of many of those correlations are not usually definitive. It is a common belief among scholars that as religious engagement increases, the likelihood of pornography consumption decreases (Nelson, Padilla-Walker, & Carroll, 2010). This may be a result of religious teaching reinforcing personal beliefs in young people about pornography; therefore, youth who practice religion are less likely to consume SEIM (Nelson et al., 2010). It is suggested that youth who abstain from Internet pornography consumption may be more engaged in their religious practice or raised by religious families (Nelson et al., 2010). The abstention from consuming Internet pornography could also be related to possible increased self-regulation and self-control that may be indicative of adolescents who practice religious rituals (Rasmussen & Bierman, 2016). Conversely, we may find that as pornography consumption increases, religious engagement decreases. For example, youth who consume Internet pornography can avoid practicing religion if they become ashamed and embarrassed if they are engaged in activity that might be labeled as sinful, immoral, or deplorable (Nelson et al., 2010).

While some religious teachings inform individuals that pornography is harmful to its very core, this does not always deter religious people from intentionally consuming Internet pornography (Nelson et al., 2010). It is possible that pornography consumption can violate one's religious doctrines but not violate one's personal beliefs (Short, Kasper, & Wetterneck, 2015). Religious individuals, regardless of what specific beliefs they hold, are still sexual beings who are living in a highly sexualized society and share the same ability to anonymously access Internet pornography (Perry, 2018). Analyses of searches on the Google search engine indicate that Internet pornography consumption may take place in more theologically conservative populated communities (Edelman, 2009; MacInnis & Hodson, 2015). Some go as far as to question if the prohibited nature of pornography encourages religious individuals to seek it out simply because its consumption is forbidden by spiritual groups (Short et al., 2015).

There is a cognitive dissonance that can occur when religious individuals consume Internet pornography. If the consumption of Internet pornography is considered a desecration of a sacred religious value, the psychological ramifications of adolescents can be substantial. For example, many adolescents with strong religious beliefs may still consume SEIM despite the message that viewing Internet pornography is an immoral act. The result may be the experience of considerable guilt, shame, and unhappiness. Religious youth who have consumed SEIM have also reported higher levels of depression and lower levels of self-worth (Nelson et al., 2010). Ultimately, negative moral feelings associated with the consumption of Internet pornography may severely impact the mental health of an adolescent. The underlying cause of cognitive dissonance may be extremely challenging for the helping professional; therefore, is it imperative that we understand the impact of such an internal conflict when a perceived moral issue clashes with an immoral one. Learning Activity 6.1 invites the reader to consider these issues in more depth.

Learning Activity 6.1

Cultural considerations in the helping process

Consider the following questions as they relate to your work as a helping professional.

1 How might an individual's age and sexual development level or sexual maturity be positively or negatively impacted by the consumption of Internet pornography?
2 Having an understanding of the biological, psychological, and social perspectives associated with gender, what impact might gender have on Internet pornography consumption?
3 What arguments can be made in support of or against the consumption of Internet pornography as a healthy and normal expression of sexuality for heterosexual and LGBTQ youth?
4 Consider your own cultural background and how your attitudes, beliefs, and behaviors have changed since your child and adolescent years?
5 How might an individual's political ideology, religious views, or worldviews influence the consumption of Internet pornography?
6 What cultural (political, religious, and worldview) values were most present in your upbringing from childhood through adolescence?

LGBTQ

As adolescents engage SEIM as part of their sexual development, viewing Internet pornography may be considered a safe space for exploring one's sexual identity outside of what is considered mainstream. The Internet has filled a cultural void by offering an endless selection of pornography with a same-sex focus, which has increased accessibility to same-sex SEIM. It has not always been the case that consumers of SEIM had access to content representative of an LGBTQ community (Poole & Milligan, 2018). SEIM with a same-sex focus, which was once considered extremely difficult to obtain, can now be easily accessed through the Internet in a matter of seconds. As a result, LGBTQ youth are significantly more likely to consume SEIM than their heterosexual peers (Træen et al., 2006) and at a much younger age (Lim, Agius, Carrotte, Vella, & Hellard, 2017).

The Internet allows many LGBTQ youth access to pornography consistent with one's sexual identity in a less restrictive environment, allowing for positive and welcoming expressions of sexual diversity. By consuming SEIM, LBGTQ youth can experience a sense of normalcy while eliminating the exposure to many of the negative stigmatizations that may be found in society (Træen et al., 2006). Consistent with their heterosexual peers, LGBTQ youth will find that SEIM can serve as a way to expand upon their sexual knowledge, attitudes, and behaviors in a safe, anonymous, and private setting. For example, youth in search of a better understanding of how to be intimate with same-sex partners may seek out SEIM as a means of education, as displays of same-sex behavior may not be widely available in their communities.

In a Swedish study (Svedin, Åkerman, & Priebe, 2011), almost all of the adolescent males interviewed reported consuming heterosexual SEIM. However, this same study found that more than half of those same participants intentionally viewed pornography consisting of sexual intercourse between same-sex partners. Many SEIM products available to consumers consist of females engaged in sexual acts with other women, and much of the consumption of this type of SEIM occurs regardless of the sexual orientation of the consumer. However, it should be noted that there also exist many individuals who identify as heterosexual who consume SEIM depicting sexual activity between males (Ross, Månsson, Daneback, & Tikkanen, 2005). For many heterosexual youth, the consumption of Internet pornography has the potential to increase the acceptance of sexual diversity and sexual open-mindedness (Hare, Gahagan, Jackson, & Steenbeek, 2014).

Conclusion

As the Internet rapidly continues to bring the entire world online, both the accidental exposure to, and deliberate consumption of, SEIM will continue to increase among adolescents. Internet pornography is more likely to be consumed as youth increase in age, and males tend to consume more SEIM than women. For both male and female youth, the viewing of pornography has come to be considered a normal behavior (Häggström-Nordin et al., 2006); however, culture will ultimately define many sexual boundaries. For many, the issue of pornography is deeply rooted in individual political ideology. Conservative thinkers are more likely to consider Internet pornography a moral issue while liberal thinkers might consider it an individual's right to free expression. It is a common belief that pornography should be a social justice issue which should be advocated in the political arena (Barker, 2014). For many seeking social justice, LGBTQ youth have found many equal opportunities with the advancement of Internet pornography and, in turn, tend to hold more positive views of consumption. For many LGBTQ youth, the consumption of Internet pornography is the only space to safely express their sexual orientation free from judgment and negative stigma.

The pornography industry continues to test the boundaries of what cultures throughout the world will consider acceptable content. After all, Intent pornography is a money-making industry, and the further it reaches, the more money it makes. Fairly consistent are worldviews and religious teachings that define sexual boundaries based on the perceived morality and overall societal impact of SEIM. Such an overwhelming negative association with sexuality may obstruct open discussions, public debate, and the quality of sex education. Many youth in non-Western cultures are less likely to consume pornography and will experience aspects of sexual development differently than their Western counterparts. For many religious youth around the world, there is a strong belief that sexually explicit content causes a breakdown in moral values.

In Learning Activity 6.2, we invite readers to bring these various cultural elements together and use their skills in active listening and interviewing to learn more about the intersection of culture and sexuality.

Learning Activity 6.2

Bringing it all together

The purposes of this exercise are (a) to provide individuals with an opportunity to reflect on the lessons they have learned about pornography from a variety of cultural influences throughout their lifetimes, (b) to provide individuals with an opportunity to practice evaluating another person around the impact of pornography on sexual development, and (c) to provide individuals with an opportunity to experience what it is like to be asked about experiences with pornography and other issues of a sexual nature in an effort to increase empathy for clients in that context.

Directions: In groups of three, one individual will be the interviewer, one individual will be the interviewee, and one individual will be the observer. You will rotate through each of these three roles. In accordance with professional ethics, group members must treat information discussed during this interview as confidential, private information. Although the information for the interviews can be fictional and role-played, it must be realistic, consistent, and based on knowledge, skill, and awareness obtained from this chapter.

To begin this exercise, the **interviewer** will ask the **interviewee** to consider pornography from a cultural perspective and to share how pornography or highly sexually explicit material has impacted his or her sexual development from childhood to adulthood. For example, relevant information pertaining to this specific assignment may include collecting information on how the following factors contributed to your role of pornography in your own sexual development: age, gender, worldview, sexual identity, political ideology, and religion. The interviewee's story should be embellished to force the interviewer to deal with difficulties related to cultural implications of pornography. The **observer** in this interview will focus on the interactions between the interviewer and the interviewee.

Before each interview, please take the time to discuss confidentiality issues with your interviewee and inform the interviewee of his or her right to not answer or ignore any question.

During the interview, please be sure to always respect the interviewee's decision regarding whether to answer or expand on a particular question. The interviewee may also bring up additional questions that he or she would like to answer or topics that he or she would like to further discuss. The aforementioned questions should only act as a guide to the interview.

After each interview, your group will meet to focus on your reactions to the process of participating in this project as the interviewer, interviewee, and observer, and not the content of the interview. You may select any of the following questions, or you may modify these questions and add additional related questions or comments.

- What was it like for you to ask the questions you asked as an interviewer?
- What was it like for you to be asked the questions you were asked as an interviewee?

84 From the self to the world

- What observations did you make as the observer related to what the process of the interview was like for the interviewer and the interviewee?
- In what ways did this interview experience help you to develop your cultural knowledge, skill, and self-awareness around Internet pornography?
- What was the most challenging aspect of participating in this interview process for you?

Summary

- As adolescents develop in a sexualized and digital society, their exposure to various types of SEIM will continue to increase. For many youth, Internet pornography will be their first introduction to sexuality and culture will be a significant factor of when and why this introduction will take place.
- As the Internet continues to grow and evolve, the availability of Internet pornography will continue to increase worldwide. For many adolescents, an increase in the availability of SEIM will likely make it difficult, if not impossible, to avoid SEIM consumption, whether intentional or unintentional.
- Older youth will likely be more deliberate in their consumption of Internet pornography and more likely to experience enjoyment than their younger peers.
- Considering youth gender differences in SEIM consumption from a social perspective, it is not uncommon for many young males to watch pornography together for reasons other than education or sexual arousal.
- When we examine consumption of SEIM from a more scientific perspective, males report seeking sexual content from Internet pornography sites at significantly higher rates than females, and males tend to increase consumption over time.
- For adolescent females, the consumption of pornography is shown to have increased over the past few decades and at a greater frequency than in previous generations.
- For many, SEIM consumption is closely related to political ideologies, and those ideologies may include strong, personally sensitive values. Significant differences in opinion, consumption, and outcomes can exist between adolescents of different ideologies.
- Culture and religion also play significant roles in the perceptions of SEIM, consumption of pornography, and results from that consumption.
- The Internet allows many LGBTQ youth access to pornography consistent with one's sexual identity in a less restrictive environment, allowing for positive and welcoming expressions of sexual diversity.

Additional resources

In print

Häggström-Nordin, E., Sandberg, J., Hanson, U., & Tydén, T. (2006). "It's everywhere!" Young Swedish people's thoughts and reflections about pornography. *Scandinavian Journal of Caring Sciences, 20*(4), 386–393. doi:10.1111/j.1471-6712.2006.00417.x

Lykke, L. C., & Cohen, P. N. (2015). The widening gender gap in opposition to pornography, 1975–2012. *Social Currents, 2*(4), 307–323. doi:10.1177/2329496515604170

On the web

Hussey, M. (2015, March). Who are the biggest consumers of online porn? *The Next Web.* Retrieved from https://thenextweb.com/market-intelligence/2015/03/24/who-are-the-biggest-consumers-of-online-porn/

Nowak, P. (2012, January). U.S. leads the way in porn production, but falls behind in profits. *Canadian Business.* Retrieved from www.canadianbusiness.com/blogs-and-comment/u-s-leads-the-way-in-porn-production-but-falls-behind-in-profits/

References

American Counseling Association. (2014). *ACA code of ethics.* Washington, DC: Author.

American Psychological Association. (2015). *APA dictionary of psychology* (2nd ed.). Washington, DC: Author.

Barker, M. (2014). Psychology and pornography: Some reflections. *Porn Studies, 1*(1–2), 120–126. doi:10.1080/23268743.2013.859468

Baumeister, R. F. (2000). Gender difference in erotic plasticity: The female sex drive as socially flexible and responsive. *Psychological Bulletin, 126*(3), 347–374. doi:10.1037/0033-2909.126.3.347

Beggan, J. K., & Allison, S. T. (2003). "What sort of man reads playboy?" The self-reported influence of playboy on the construction of masculinity. *The Journal of Men's Studies, 11*(2), 189–206. doi:10.3149/jms.1102.189

Behun, R. J., Cerrito, J. A., Delmonico, D. L., & Campenni, C. E. (2017). Curricular abstinence: Examining human sexuality training in school counselor preparation programs. *Journal of School Counseling, 15*(14). Retrieved from www.jsc.montana.edu/articles/v15n14.pdf

Bleakley, A., Hennessy, M., & Fishbein, M. (2011). A model of adolescents' seeking of sexual content in their media choices. *Journal of Sex Research, 48*(4), 309–315. doi:10.1080/00224499.2010.497985

Cooper, D. T., & Klein, J. L. (2017). College students' online pornography use: Contrasting general and specific structural variables with social learning variables. *American Journal of Criminal Justice, 43*(3), 551–569. doi:10.1007/s12103-017-9424-4

Diamond, M. (2009). Pornography, public acceptance and sex related crime: A review. *International Journal of Law and Psychiatry, 32*(5), 304–314. doi:10.1016/j.ijlp.2009.06.004

Edelman, B. (2009). Markets: Red light states: Who buys online adult entertainment? *Journal of Economic Perspectives, 23*, 209–220. doi:10.1257/jep.23.1.209

Frutos, A. M., & Merrill, R. M. (2017). Explicit sexual movie viewing in the United States according to selected marriage and lifestyle, work and financial, religion and political factors. *Sexuality & Culture: An Interdisciplinary Quarterly, 21*(4), 1062–1082. doi:10.1007/s12119-017-9438-6

Häggström-Nordin, E., Sandberg, J., Hanson, U., & Tydén, T. (2006). "It's everywhere!" Young Swedish people's thoughts and reflections about pornography. *Scandinavian Journal of Caring Sciences, 20*(4), 386–393. doi:10.1111/j.1471-6712.2006.00417.x

Hald, G., & Malamuth, N. (2008). Self-perceived effects of pornography consumption. *Archives of Sexual Behavior, 37*(4), 614–625. doi:10.1007/s10508-007-9212-1

Hare, K., Gahagan, J., Jackson, L., & Steenbeek, A. (2014). Perspectives on "pornography": Exploring sexually explicit internet movies' influences on Canadian young adults' holistic sexual health. *Canadian Journal of Human Sexuality, 23*(3), 148–158. doi:10.3138/cjhs.2732

Lim, M. S. C., Agius, P. A., Carrotte, E. R., Vella, A. M., & Hellard, M. E. (2017). Young Australians' use of pornography and associations with sexual risk behaviors. *Sexual Health, 41*(4), 438–443. doi:10.1111/1753-6405.12678

Lykke, L. C., & Cohen, P. N. (2015). The widening gender gap in opposition to pornography, 1975–2012. *Social Currents, 2*(4), 307–323. doi:10.1177/2329496515604170

Ma, C. M. S., & Shek, D. T. L. (2013). Consumption of pornographic materials in early adolescents in Hong Kong. *Journal of Pediatric and Adolescent Gynecology, 26*(3), 518–525. doi:10.1016/j.jpag.2013.03.011

MacInnis, C. C., & Hodson, G. (2015). Do American states with more religious or conservative populations search more for sexual content on Google? *Archives of Sexual Behavior, 44*(1), 137–147. doi:10.1007/s10508-014-0361-8

Mohd Azizuddin, M. S. (2011). Cultural arguments against offensive speech in Malaysia: Debates between liberalism and Asian values on pornography and hate speech. *Mediterranean Journal of Social Sciences, 2*(2), 122–134.

Nelson, L. J., Padilla-Walker, L. M., & Carroll, J. S. (2010). "I believe it is wrong but I still do it": A comparison of religious young males who do versus do not use pornography. *Psychology of Religion and Spirituality, 2*(3), 136–147. doi:10.1037/a0019127

Patterson, R., & Price, J. (2012). Pornography, religion, and the happiness gap: Does pornography impact the actively religious differently? *Journal for the Scientific Study of Religion, 51*(1), 79–89. doi:10.1111/j.1468-5906.2011.01630.x

Perry, S. L. (2018). Not practicing what you preach: Religion and incongruence between pornography beliefs and usage. *Journal of Sex Research, 55*(3), 369–380. doi:10.1080/00224499.2017.1333569

Perry, S. L., & Schleifer, C. (2017). Race and trends in pornography viewership, 1973–2016: Examining the moderating roles of gender and religion. *Journal of Sex Research, 56*(1), 62–73. doi:10.1080/00224499.2017.1404959

Poole, J., & Milligan, R. (2018). Nettersexuality: The impact of internet pornography on gay male sexual expression and identity. *Sexuality & Culture: An Interdisciplinary Quarterly, 22*(4), 1189–1204. doi:10.1007/s12119-018-9521-7

Rasmussen, K., & Bierman, A. (2016). How does religious attendance shape trajectories of pornography use across adolescence? *Journal of Adolescence, 49*, 191–203. doi:10.1016/j.adolescence.2016.03.017

Ross, M. W., Månsson, S. A., Daneback, K., & Tikkanen, R. (2005). Characteristics of males who have sex with males on the internet but identify as heterosexual, compared with heterosexually identified males who have sex with women. *Cyber Psychology & Behavior, 8*(2), 131–139. doi:10.1089/cpb.2005.8.131

Short, M. B., Kasper, T. E., & Wetterneck, C. T. (2015). The relationship between religiosity and internet pornography use. *Journal of Religion and Health, 54*(2), 571–583. doi:10.1007/s10943-014-9849-8

Svedin, C. G., Åkerman, I., & Priebe, G. (2011). Frequent users of pornography: A population based epidemiological study of Swedish male adolescents. *Journal of Adolescence*, *34*(4), 779–788. doi:10.1016/j.adolescence.2010.04.010

Træen, B., Nilsen, T. S., & Stigum, H. (2006). Use of pornography in traditional media and on the internet in Norway. *Journal of Sex Research*, *43*(3), 245–254. doi:10.1080/00224490609552323

Tsaliki, L. (2011). Playing with porn: Greek children's explorations in pornography. *Sex Education*, *11*(3), 293–302. doi:10.1080/14681811.2011.590087

Willoughby, B. J., Carroll, J. S., Nelson, L. J., & Padilla-Walker, L. M. (2014). Associations between relational sexual behaviour, pornography use, and pornography acceptance among US college students. *Culture, Health & Sexuality*, *16*(9), 1052–1069. doi:10.1080/13691058.2014.927075

7 Potential pitfalls

Legal and ethical issues in the field

> I worry a lot about working with adolescents, especially when it comes to the law and ethics. Legal issues have always scared me, and ethics are so complicated. It's hard to know what to do sometimes and then mix in sexuality. Mix in pornography . . . and the Internet. I'm not sure what's legal and what's not. I'm not sure what I should be telling my client's guardians. I don't even know how I feel about all of this. I know as a parent, there are things I would never want my kids doing online, and my clients are doing those very things. I want to tell their parents because I'd want to know if it was me . . . but can I?

As technology advances at breakneck speeds, helping professionals are challenged to keep up with the changes. What makes it more difficult, as evidenced by the vignette, are the ethical and legal ramifications of those advances in technology. Working with adolescents is never easy and addressing issues of sexuality with clients young or old can be difficult. However, when we think about the legal and ethical ramifications of the issues, it can become overwhelming.

When considering the intersection of Internet pornography with ethical and legal issues related to this population, helping professionals have a responsibility to act in the best interest of their clients while respecting laws, rules, regulations, and applicable ethical standards. To better understand this responsibility, the legal and ethical focus of this chapter is twofold. First, this chapter will address ethical issues and the obligations for helping professionals who work with adolescents who consume Internet pornography. Second, this chapter will examine the legal issues and obligations for helping professionals who are mandated to protect children from harm. After reading this chapter, you should be able to

1. Understand that, above all else, the primary responsibility of the helping professional is to protect and promote the welfare of the adolescent client;
2. Know the importance of ethical codes in the helping professions and the fundamental principles of professional ethical behavior;
3. Have a general understanding of laws that were designed to regulate the production, dissemination, and consumption of SEIM;
4. Identify ethical dilemmas regarding the production, dissemination, and consumption of SEIM and apply an ethical decision-making model;

5   Be knowledgeable about the impacts of child sexual abuse and understand how personal values, attitudes, and beliefs can influence a practitioner's ethical decision-making process; and
6   Consider the future of Internet pornography in an increasingly sexually permissive society and what impact philosophical arguments may have on the future of Internet pornography laws.

Ethics, law, and pornography

The legal and ethical debate regarding sexuality is not a new one. Being deeply rooted in morality and religion, people have been encouraged to flee from sexuality. However, not all individuals consider sexuality to be a moral issue. Many consider sexuality to be a basic human right and SEIM to be a freedom of expression. Regardless of the philosophical differences, a fairly consistent agreement has been that separate laws should exist for adults (individuals over the age of 18) and minors (youth who have not yet reached adulthood or at least the age of 18) regardless of one's physical, psychological, or sexual development. The common belief is that minors may be unable and incapable of always making competent sexual decisions and are more vulnerable than adults. If one accepts this premise, then it follows that extra precautions ensuring the safety of minors are warranted.

Many sexual freedoms enjoyed by adults are not always considered acceptable sexual freedoms permissible for minors. For example, many countries allow youth to consent to sexual intercourse prior to reaching adulthood but prohibit minors from legally consenting to participate in pornography. With the intention of protecting minors from harm, governments have enacted laws based on what is believed to be morally justifiable and in the best interest of youth. Ethical practitioners share that same philosophical belief in that their primary obligation is to protect and promote the welfare of their clients.

With technological advancements introducing sexuality into the digital age, the morally charged issue of SEIM, combined with the obligation to protect minors from harm, has created a plethora of unexpected ethical and legal challenges for helping professionals. The purpose of this chapter is to give the reader a balanced and unbiased overview of the ethical and legal issues related to helping professionals and youth consumers of Internet pornography.

Ethical issues and obligations for helping professionals

Ethics define the helping professions by providing practitioners with a philosophical and moral framework by which to practice. Through a series of codified standards, ethical codes are created by professional organizations to help guide its members in practicing the highest standard of moral and ethical conduct. These codes are designed to hold helping professionals to the highest levels of professional integrity but also hold helping professionals accountable when unethical conduct occurs. A violation of an ethical code may result in censure or dismissal from a professional organization or loss of credential. Not only do these codes guide the ethical practice of helping professionals, but they also educate the public on a set of commonly held beliefs, values, and principles put in place that are designed to protect client welfare.

As the options for selecting professional membership seems somewhat endless for practitioners, it does become just as much a personal decision as a professional one. The same could be said for selecting ethical codes to follow. Helping professionals have an obligation to understand and follow the specific ethical codes as defined by the professional organizations in which they are members. For the purposes of this book, the ACA Code of Ethics (2014) will be highlighted to help guide this chapter. The ACA represents professional counselors who work in a plethora of settings.

Moral principles

In addition to its Code of Ethics, the ACA (2014) defines six moral principles of professional ethical behavior that all helping professionals could follow. These fundamental principles of professional ethical behavior are autonomy, nonmaleficence, beneficence, justice, fidelity, and veracity. Practitioners may promote client ***autonomy*** by respecting the independence of the youth who are ultimately free to make many life decisions. Helping professionals who respect autonomy are nonjudgmental practitioners who do not impose their own values on their youth clients. ***Nonmaleficence*** simply means, above all else, do no harm. Being mindful of both intentional and unintentional causes of harm, helping professionals who practice nonmaleficence avoid any action that may place their clients at-risk of experiencing harm. Professionals practicing ***beneficence*** should work for the good of the client by promoting positive mental health and overall wellness. Beneficence may extend beyond individual clients if the need is for the betterment of society.

Justice involves treating individuals equitably. By fostering fairness, equality, and impartiality, helping professionals must ensure that all clients are given the same quality of service and access to treatment. In the helping professions, ***fidelity*** refers to practitioners keeping promises and honoring commitments to clients. For example, fidelity could be promoted by maintaining confidentiality in a therapeutic relationship. Honoring fidelity will allow for trust to develop and helps establish a safe environment for the client. Lastly, helping professionals must be truthful and honest with their clients through the practice of ***veracity*** . Practicing veracity will show genuineness and will further strengthen trust within the therapeutic relationship, ultimately allowing clients to become vulnerable and more open to personal growth.

Ethical responsibility to youth

Above all else, the primary responsibility of the helping professional is to protect and promote the welfare of the youth client (ACA, 2014, Standard A.1.a.). This ethical standard is not taken lightly and should be prioritized at all times by the ethical helping professional. However, maintaining confidentiality in the therapeutic setting does come with its limitations, especially when working with sensitive topics. When considering the limitations of confidentiality, helping professionals may be required to breach confidentiality consistent with legal requirements or in light of other ethical considerations. For example, as mandated by most laws, helping professionals are required to report instances when youth disclose forms of abuse, including sexual abuse. When working with youth clients who are in treatment related to the consumption of Internet pornography, the likelihood of a disclosure that would require a mandated report is always a possibility. As the topic of mandated reporting will be discussed in greater depth later in this chapter, it should be noted that the ethical responsibility of breaching confidentiality comes at the potential expense of a loss of trust in the therapeutic relationship if not done appropriately.

Recognizing that trust is the cornerstone of any therapeutic relationship, counselors and other professionals are responsible for protecting the confidentiality of their clients' disclosures and information. An ethical practitioner makes it clear through a process of informed consent that such confidential information is only disclosed to a third party in very rare cases and only when required. However, it can be difficult for practitioners to maintain that confidentiality when parents or other guardians do not completely understand the importance of confidentiality. For example, most legal jurisdictions recognize the natural right of the parent or guardian to be active participants in the welfare of the child. Guided by ethical principles, helping professionals must respect these inherent rights, be sensitive to the cultural diversity of families, and work to establish collaborative relationships with parents or guardians (ACA, 2014, Standard B.5.b).

Personal values

Personal beliefs have the potential to impact the therapeutic relationship if helping professionals are unaware of their own beliefs or biases. Ethical practitioners must be aware of, and avoid imposing, their own personal values, beliefs, and attitudes on to their clients (ACA, 2014, Standard A.4.b.). When conflicts in values do arise, practitioners should refer to the professional values or practice policies of their professional organizations (e.g., ACA, American Psychological Association, National Association of Social Workers). Helping professionals can also find a great deal of guidance by seeking consultation with another practitioner or supervisor.

Boundaries of competence

A lack of training in human sexuality may compel practitioners to rely on their own personal beliefs as opposed to proper knowledge, skill, and self-awareness (Behun, Cerrito, Delmonico, & Campenni, 2017). Helping professionals must practice within the boundaries of their competence by only practicing in areas in which they were educated or trained or have had supervised experience (ACA, 2014, Standard C.2.a). Most culturally competent helping professionals should be able to ethically work with a diverse client population, such as youth who have been impacted by the consumption of Internet pornography. However, practitioners should continue their professional development in order to strengthen their competencies in an area as sensitive and personal as sexuality.

Research with youth participants

Helping professionals who wish to contribute to the knowledge base of adolescent consumption of SEIM must conduct research in accordance with ethical codes, laws, Institutional Review Board policies, and other scientific standards (ACA, 2014, Standard G.1.a). It is highly recommended that researchers who work with youth complete research ethics and compliance training prior to engaging in any such endeavor. Conducting research with youth who consume SEIM can create many unique challenges and may not even be permissible in all jurisdictions. Helping professionals conducting research in this area are working with a vulnerable population that may not be developmentally mature enough to fully comprehend the personal risk associated with sexuality research. For this reason, many Institutional Review Boards will require the implementation of protective measures before approving any such study.

Much like the ethical obligations helping professionals owe to youth clients, researchers must follow similar requirements related to informed consent and confidentiality when conducting research. It is the obligation of the helping professional to weigh the potential risks associated with Internet pornography research against potential benefits prior to inviting youth to participate. Ultimately, it is the highest responsibility of the researcher to protect a young participant from any potential risk by taking reasonable precautions to avoid causing emotional, physical, or social harm (ACA, 2014, Standard G.1.e.).

Laws and legal issues and obligations for helping professionals

In addition to ethical codes, it is of the utmost importance that helping professionals are knowledgeable about the local laws and regulations applicable to practicing in their jurisdictions (ACA, 2014). In an ideal world, ethical codes and laws would be consistent with one another, leaving little room for disagreement. However, this is not always the case, and laws and ethical codes occasionally deviate from one another. For the ethical practitioner, it is of the utmost importance to understand that when conflicts between ethical codes and laws exist, helping professionals must always act in the best interest of their clients. In these rare circumstances, helping professionals should advocate that professional ethical codes be followed but may ultimately need to adhere to the law (ACA, 2014, Standard I.1.c.). In other words, laws trump ethics.

Laws are different from ethical codes in that these rules and regulations are designed for all of society, are established by the government, and a violation of such laws may result in fines or imprisonment. As different countries have different forms of government, mores, norms, and so forth, local laws are often consistent with varying worldviews and may vary widely. Regarding the Internet, pornography laws will vary greatly around the world. While these laws do have some similarities, it would be an impossible task to explore each specific law in every country or local jurisdiction. Therefore, this chapter will aim to capture a general legal understanding of various laws related to Internet pornography.

Internet pornography laws could be created as proactive or reactive measures. A legislative branch of government could pass a law with the intent of preventing future production, dissemination, or consumption of SEIM. For example, in an attempt to restrict children from accessing pornography websites online, the United Kingdom has passed the Digital Economy Act (2017). The Digital Economy Act requires Internet pornography websites to verify consumers are at least 18 years old before accessing sexually explicit content. It is also common to see reactive measures passed in the form of case law. Judicial branches of government have the ability to interpret laws and set legal precedent. For example, the current legal standard for pornography was established by the United States Supreme Court in *Miller v. California* in 1973, long before the existence of the World Wide Web and Internet pornography.

Philosophical legal arguments

There are two fairly common legal arguments made regarding the regulation of Internet pornography. Perhaps the most common argument made in favor of Internet pornography is the right to free expression or free speech. In other words, many believe that the ability to view consenting adults engaged in sexually explicit conduct online is a basic human right. Opponents have generally argued that Internet pornography is immoral, sinful, and is harmful to society. However, from a legal perspective, a common belief of both supporters and opponents of Internet pornography is that the potential risk and impact for harm is significantly greater when children are the consumer.

Unprotected free speech and expression

For minors, many laws consider Internet pornography harmful to youth, making its production, dissemination, and consumption illegal. However, this is not the case for adults. For many adults, the production, dissemination, and consumption of Internet pornography is generally considered a protected type of sexual expression under the law and is completely legal. Although the freedom of sexual expression is extended to all adults, that freedom does not go completely unchecked and does have limitations. For example, many laws regulating the freedom of sexual expression will limit SEIM that is morally unacceptable according to community standards. Regardless of the Internet pornography consumer's age, there are two notable categories of pornography that are not considered protected free speech or expression and are outright banned: obscenity (Miller v. California, 1973) and child pornography (New York v. Ferber, 1982).

Regarding obscene pornography, obscenity laws exist throughout the world and are meant to place limitations on some sexually explicit material that may be deemed immoral or especially harmful to society. For example, Canadian law regards obscene sexual acts involving crime, horror, cruelty, or violence to be a corruption of morals (Criminal Code, 1985). Additionally, the Obscene Publications Act (1959) in the United Kingdom and the *Miller* test in the United States both define obscenity and lay a foundation of determining harm. For example, the *Miller* test gives society a reasonable person standard for determining if sexually explicit material is patently offensive under contemporary community standards and lacking serious literary, artistic, political or scientific value (Miller v. California, 1973). Some extreme "hardcore" pornography may be limited if considered outright harmful to society. However, this community standard was created long before the digital age and without the Internet as a consideration. What was once extremely difficult to judge or define at a local level has evolved into an unrealistic standard as the Internet reaches beyond local legal jurisdictions.

Helping professionals should understand that youth are in a more vulnerable place in the world and, therefore, are a protected class. The standards applied to adults may differ from the standard applied to minors. Therefore, helping professionals must consider how obscene pornographic material may be harmful to minors and what laws are in place specifically designed to protect youth. For example, U.S. laws prohibit using misleading domain names (18 U.S.C. §2252B) or embedding words or digital images (18 U.S.C. §2252C) with the intent to deceive an adolescent into viewing material that is obscene or harmful to minors. Other laws prohibit the dissemination of obscene material and increase the penalty when such material is shared with a minor.

Regarding child pornography, laws exist to protect children from sexual abuse and minors cannot legally be depicted in pornographic material (New York v. Ferber, 1982). Child pornography is considered an unacceptable and illegal practice throughout nearly the entire world. In addition, because child pornography laws are intended to protect vulnerable children from exploitation, these laws are rarely challenged. In the United States, child pornography is defined as

> any visual depiction, including any photograph, film, video, picture, or computer or computer-generated image or picture, whether made or produced by electronic, mechanical, or other means, of sexually explicit conduct, where (A) the production of such visual depiction involves the use of a minor engaging in sexually explicit conduct; (B) such visual depiction is a digital image, computer image, or computer-generated image that is, or is indistinguishable from, that of a minor engaging in sexually explicit conduct; or (C) such visual depiction has been created, adapted, or modified to appear that an identifiable minor is engaging in sexually explicit conduct.
>
> (18 U.S.C. §2256)

While this is considered a criminal offense with significant penalties including fines and imprisonment, the production, dissemination, and possession of child pornography continues to be a reality.

From a legal standpoint, laws exist that require production companies to verify the age of a pornography actor or actress prior to filming (Child Protection and Obscenity Act, 1988). However, in an attempt to legally accommodate a child pornography market, producers aim to employ adult actors and actresses who look young, as if they were minors. It may be extremely difficult for anyone to know the difference between a pornography actor or actress who is 17 (illegal) or 18 (legal). In an effort to create pornography that is legal but still depicts adolescents engaged in sexual activity, adults can intentionally look to be underage and could be indistinguishable from minors.

Advancements in technology and the law

Another way to legally accommodate a child pornography market is though advances in technology. Technological advances have allowed for the creation of computer-generated (i.e., not real) images of children engaged in sexually explicit conduct, essentially resulting in a virtual type of child pornography. At this point in the digital age, imaging technology has advanced to the point where it is nearly impossible for many to distinguish between real and virtual pornographic images (see the chapter on current issues for more about *deepfake* technology). The completely digital image of a "child" engaging in sexually explicit conduct may disgust the majority of individuals, but this production does not require or involve an actual child. Although the appearance of child pornography is present, no actual child is sexually harmed in the production of this type of digital imagery. Therefore, computer-generated images that do not involve children in their production are not legally considered child pornography in the United States (Ashcroft v. Free Speech Coalition, 2002).

Much of the Internet pornography found around the world is produced and disseminated with little outside regulation or government oversight. Countries around the world have little or no control over where Internet pornography is generated or distributed. The only preventive measure that can be taken in addition to failed legal deterrents is to attempt to combat consumption through the use of technology. Accountability systems, such as blocking, filtering, and monitoring software, can be installed on devices with Internet access; however, such technology is not completely failsafe (Behun, Sweeney, Delmonico, & Griffin, 2012). Because the Internet is worldwide, SEIM can be produced and disseminated in one country and consumed in another, making regulation extremely difficult. With the lack of a mechanism to ensure that the potential consumer of Internet pornography is of a legal viewing age, the decision to enter a pornographic site online relies solely on the "honor system" of the adolescent. Almost any young person can search the Internet unchecked; limiting access or increasing accountability may be easier said than done.

A major legal consideration is how archaic laws are applied to current legal issues pertaining to SEIM. As the Internet has quickly expanded throughout the world, it has been impossible to simultaneously create laws regulating its use. Technological advancements are fast moving, ever changing, and relatively immediate; conversely, the system of creating, debating, passing, and implementing laws is slow. It is likely possible that the law will never be able to keep up with the growing pace of the Internet or the supply and demand of SEIM. With the unpredictable advances in technology, lawmakers and helping professionals alike will continue to be challenged with the desire for developing adolescents to test the boundaries of sexuality in the digital age.

Sexting

An often-overlooked means of producing, distributing, receiving, and consuming child pornography is through the use of mobile devices and smartphones. For many youth, creating sexually explicit photos or videos and electronically sharing with others has become a phenomenon made possible by cellular or wireless Internet connections. Through a practice known as "sexting," just about anyone with a cellular phone can become an amateur producer of pornography. Similarly, any minor who can upload that same video to the Internet can also instantly become a distributor.

When we consider the free sexual expression of consenting adults, sexting can be considered a responsible practice meant to enhance a sexual relationship; however, it is almost always considered harmful when practiced by minors. Sexting can carry with it numerous criminal and civil law issues for minors if obscenity and child pornography laws are being violated. Minors who send messages containing sexual images of other minors are exploiting a vulnerable population (Wolak & Finkelhor, 2011) and can potentially be violating child pornography laws.

Sexting photos and videos of minors engaged in sexually explicit conduct does not always stop with the intended recipient. For example, a sext message from one youth to another could easily turn into a group discussion. Sexting can be intended to be flirtatious; it can also be intended to harm. For example, a current issue with sexting is when it is used to shame another individual through a means known as "revenge porn." Revenge porn is when an individual shares sexually explicit images of another individual in order to humiliate, harass, or seek revenge and is a violation of a basic human right (FindLaw, 2019). Having an intimate photo or video intended for a romantic partner shared among a circle of peers or online for the world to consume could have a detrimental psychological impact on a youth.

Although considered illegal and harmful to youth, confusion often exists for the mandated reporter when the perpetrator and victim of sexual abuse are both minors (Behun & Cerrito, 2016). For example, many mandated reporters are expecting to report a stereotypical adult pedophile engaging in child pornography. Helping professionals must also report when minors are engaged in child pornography, as the seriousness of the crime warrants legal involvement for the protection of children. When such harmful and illegal instances of sexting do get reported, minors who might not usually be treated as adults will be in the same situation. It is possible that a minor will not be prosecuted for a child pornography offense unless another element such as sexual exploitation, extortion, or harassment also exist (Slane, 2013).

Mandated reporting

It is important for helping professionals to understand the legal issues related to pornography as some client disclosures may result in what is called a "mandated report." *Mandated reporting* is required across the United States and in many other jurisdictions; it is the legal requirement that a helping professional report child abuse to the authorities. In some jurisdictions, minors responsible for producing digital content depicting oneself or other minors engaging in sexually explicit conduct may have engaged in child sexual abuse. For example, this might include a sexually explicit cell phone video being shared via social media. For many mandated reporters, disclosure of the digital production, dissemination, or consumption of minors engaged in sexually explicit acts would constitute a violation of child pornography laws.

Helping professionals are rarely the direct witnesses to child sexual abuse and typically only report what was disclosed by a client; however, the decision to report can be a difficult one to make (Behun, Owens, & Cerrito, 2015). Possibly the most common reason helping professionals will not report suspected child sexual abuse is because they believe they lack sufficient evidence to be completely positive that a child was victimized (Behun, Cerrito, Delmonico, & Kolbert, 2019). Helping professionals must be aware of the local laws regulating the degree of certainty required to make a mandated report, the protections offered for making a report in good faith, and the penalties for failing to report.

Regardless of the criminal or civil penalties for failure to make a mandated report of child sexual abuse, helping professionals sometimes elect not to file a report for personal reasons (Behun et al., 2019). For example, mandated reporters may fear legal consequences for making an unfounded report. They may believe a report will cause the child more harm than good or lack confidence in child protective services taking the report. They may also fear retaliation from the abuser (Behun et al., 2017). In addition, a topic as sensitive as child sexual abuse (e.g., child pornography) may cause the helping professional to feel significant discomfort and avoidance may become an easy defense mechanism. Helping professionals must continue to examine the personal impacts of child sexual abuse and understand that mandated reporting is meant to help protect the youth for which they are ethically and legally responsible (Behun et al., 2019).

Conclusion

The morally charged issue of Internet pornography and the obligation to protect minors from harm will likely continue to create ethical and legal challenges for helping professionals. When working with adolescent consumers of SEIM, helping professionals have fundamental moral principles and professional ethical codes to help guide them toward accepted best practice. Ethical standards guide helping professionals to practice an ideal model of conduct.

At the heart of many legal documents is the recognition that minors are a vulnerable population and are in need of greater protections. This increased legal standard of care becomes one of the greatest responsibilities bestowed upon the helping professional. Specific to the government interest in preventing minors from engaging in the production, dissemination, and consumption of Internet pornography, helping professionals must understand that the most significant function of these laws is to protect children. Misunderstanding an ethical responsibility or unknowingly violating a local law or regulation can result in a charge of unethical behavior or illegal conduct. To practice both ethically and legally, helping professionals must have a heightened self-awareness of their own attitudes, values, and beliefs regarding SEIM and the adolescents who consume it.

Having read the chapter, Learning Activity 7.1 provides you with an opportunity to practice what you have learned through the application of an ethical decision-making model on a case illustration.

> ### Learning Activity 7.1
>
> **The case of Teddy**
>
> When helping professionals are faced with an ethical dilemma that is difficult to resolve, ethical practitioners are expected to apply an ethical decision-making model as a course of action. There are many of these models, and none are considered more effective than another; however, helping professionals must follow a credible model of decision making that can bear public scrutiny (ACA, 2014). The purpose of this exercise is to provide individuals with an opportunity to implement an ethical decision-making model by (a) applying an ethical code and the moral principles to and ethical dilemma, (b) seeking consultation and considering self-awareness through an evaluation of personal feelings, and (c) considering the cultural context of the dilemma and how the client should be involved in the ethical decision-making process. Upon completing these critical steps, you will determine the best course of action to resolve your ethical dilemma.
>
> **Directions:** Read the following case study and then apply the elements of the comprehensive ethical decision-making model that follows (presented in the *ACA Ethical Standards Casebook* (Herlihy & Corey, 2015).
>
> You are a mental health counselor at a rural high school in the United States. Teddy is a 16-year-old Caucasian, heterosexual male who is a junior at your school and on your caseload. His parents are conservative, religious, well-known, and respected members of the community. Teddy is an outstanding student and has recently been recognized as an Eagle Scout by the Boy Scouts of America. Each day, Teddy boards a school bus, joined by other high school and middle school students for a long, and rather boring, ride to school. During the morning commute, students on the bus normally sleep or study in preparation for the day's classes. During the afternoon commute home, students are generally more alert and socially active.
>
> Numerous times last week, parents have complained to the school administration about rumors that a boy named Teddy was using his cell phone

to video record eighth-grade girls in the back of the school bus who were believed to have exposed their breasts. In fact, one parent claimed that a girl was filmed performing oral sex on Teddy, which was later posted online. It is believed that numerous students have witnessed these acts. At this point, school administrators began an investigation.

The supervisor of transportation and the bus driver were notified that the audio and video recordings from the school bus would need to be downloaded and forwarded to administration to aid in the investigation. In compliance with the administration's request, the bus driver downloaded the recordings and aired the recordings on the breakroom monitor, which was viewed by numerous other bus drivers and the supervisor of transportation. To their astonishment, the rumors were justified; Teddy had engaged in sexually explicit conduct with an eighth-grade girl while recording the entire event on his phone.

The supervisor at the bus garage confirmed that the rumored video existed by emailing the video to all district administrators who were able to see Teddy engaged in sexually explicit conduct while filming the entire act. Administrators immediately confiscated Teddy's phone and asked him to show the video he recorded on the bus. Teddy, afraid of expulsion, complied with the school administration, who demanded the video be immediately deleted. Teddy informed the school administration that the video could be deleted from his phone, but it already had been shared through text message with numerous other boys in the junior class who may have it saved. In addition, Teddy informed administrators that the video had already been uploaded to an online pornography website.

School administrators agreed that both students' parents should be notified that their children had engaged in sexually explicit conduct on the bus and a video was recorded on a student's phone, which has since been deleted. Being such a close-knit, religious, and rural community, neither the parents nor the school administration wanted the embarrassment of a sexual scandal.

You are very well aware that this incident was not reported by school administration at the request of the parents and understand that if this incident were to be reported to authorities, it would eventually be made public. At the request of the involved parents and the administration, you will begin meeting with Teddy several times a week to provide counseling. Although you have not personally witnessed the video from the bus or Teddy's videos, you understand that they exist and know what has taken place on both recordings. You know that multiple adults intentionally watched the video before sharing it with numerous adults who knew that the video could contain sexually explicit images of minors. In addition, other recordings of the same sexually explicit act saved on Teddy's phone were intentionally viewed by school administrators. You know that the video was shared and viewed among several minors and that a copy of the video exists online.

With your understanding of the law, you believe that the video produced by Teddy and could be considered child pornography. In addition, you believe that even though their intentions may not have been bad, multiple school employees and administrators viewed and shared this video through email. As an ethical practitioner, you feel strongly that that local law enforcement should have been involved in this situation from the beginning and that a child sexual abuse report should be filed in accordance with your duties as a mandated reporter. However, there is a conflict between your professional obligations as a mandated reporter and your personal feelings that a report could potentially cause more harm and prevent a positive therapeutic relationship with Teddy.

On one hand, if you are able to establish rapport with Teddy, you may be able to help him and possibly prevent a similar incident from happening again. This may ultimately prevent harm to another young female in the future. On the other hand, fulfilling your legal obligation may cause Teddy and his family a significant amount of embarrassment, shame, and disgust in the community. You know that it would be extremely difficult for you to establish any type of trust or rapport with Teddy once his behavior was reported to authorities.

As you consider the ethics of this case, use the following model to attempt to resolve the dilemma:

- *Identify the problem*. After reading the scenario, identify and list any and all legal and ethical issues that may arise. For the purpose of this activity, just focus on the ethical issues from this point forward.
- *Examine the relevant codes of ethics and the professional literature*. Using an ethics code of your choice, examine the code for any and all applicable standards that may be useful in addressing the ethical issues you just have identified. If possible, additional literature can be referenced at this point to help address the issues.
- *Consider the moral principles*. Consider the moral principles of autonomy, nonmaleficence, beneficence, justice, fidelity, and veracity. How might each of these fundamental principles of professional ethical behavior apply to this case?
- *Consult with colleagues, supervisors, or experts*. After identifying the ethical issues and applying the ethical codes and moral principles, have a colleague read over the scenario. Once your colleague has reviewed the scenario, consult with your colleague to review any the presenting ethical issues. This will ensure that you are meeting a professional legal standard of conduct and have considered all possible ethical issues.
- *Attend to your emotions*. Considering that your own self-awareness is equally important as having the knowledge and skill to address an ethical dilemma, now is the time to consider any emotions you are having about the case. Feel free to discuss your personal feelings after initially reading the case and after your consultation with your colleague and determine how you might feel moving forward. At this step in the process, you should recognize how your own personal values, beliefs, and attitudes might be present and influence the ethical decision-making process.

- *Involve your client in the decision-making process.* Although your client has been a consideration the entire time you have been going through the steps, make it a point to empower your client by involving the individual in the ethical decision-making process as much as possible.
- *Consider the cultural context.* Helping professionals must understand that a client's culture or worldview may differ from their own. In this case, you may need to educate yourself on a new cultural perspective by either doing your own research or engaging your client in a conversation about values. It can also be helpful to seek additional consultation from a colleague who has experience with a culture similar to your client's.
- *Identify, evaluate, and implement your selected course of action.* Consider as many courses of action as possible and review these potential outcomes with a colleague. If you and a colleague are in agreement on the best way to approach resolving your ethical dilemma, you will have one more point to consider before implementing your plan. It is of the utmost importance that you are absolutely certain, knowing that the course of action you are implementing will be the same course of action another competent helping professional, who you believe will always practice an ideal model of conduct, would implement in a similar situation. Once you are certain you have fulfilled the legal duty owed to your client, your final step is to implement your plan.

Summary

- When considering the intersection of Internet pornography with ethical and legal issues related to this population, helping professionals have a responsibility to act in the best interest of their clients while respecting laws, rules, regulations, and applicable ethical standards.
- Regardless of the philosophical differences, a fairly consistent agreement has been that separate laws should exist for adults (individuals over the age of 18) and minors (youth who have not yet reached adulthood or at least the age of 18).
- With technological advancements introducing sexuality into the digital age, the morally charged issue of SEIM, combined with the obligation to protect minors from harm, has created a plethora of unexpected ethical and legal challenges for helping professionals.
- Through a series of codified standards, ethical codes are created by professional organizations to help guide its members in practicing the highest standard of moral and ethical conduct. Violation of ethical codes can result in censure or dismissal from a professional organization and loss of professional credentials.

- The ACA identifies six moral principles of ethical behavior: autonomy, nonmaleficence, beneficence, justice, fidelity, and veracity.
- When considering work with young people, confidentiality may not be able to be maintained given legal and ethical considerations; however, helping professionals should attempt, whenever possible, to maintain the confidence of clients to promote the therapeutic relationship.
- Ethical practitioners must be aware of, and avoid imposing, their own personal values, beliefs, and attitudes on to their clients.
- Laws are different from ethical codes in that the former are rules and regulations designed for all of society and established by the government; a violation of such laws may result in fines or imprisonment.
- There are two common legal arguments regarding SEIM: one involves free speech rights; the other involves the protection of society from harm. Limits exist to any free speech argument, most notably limits related to obscenity and child pornography.
- Technological advancements are fast moving, ever changing, and relatively immediate; conversely, the system of creating, debating, passing, and implementing laws is slow.
- Mandated reporting is the legal requirement that a helping professional report child abuse to the authorities.

Additional resources

In print

Behun, R. J., & Cerrito, J. A. (2016). Defining child abuse for professional counselors as mandated reporters in Pennsylvania under the newly amended Child Protective Services Law. *Journal of the Pennsylvania Counseling Association, 15*(1), 39–43.

Herlihy, B., & Corey, G. (2015). *ACA ethical standards casebook* (7th ed.). Alexandria, VA: ACA.

On the web

American Counseling Association. (2014). *ACA code of ethics*. Alexandria, VA: Author. Retrieved from www.counseling.org/resources/aca-code-of-ethics.pdf

Wolak, J., & Finkelhor, D. (2011, March). Sexting: A typology. *Crimes Against Children Research Center Bulletin*. Retrieved from www.unh.edu/ccrc/pdf/CV231_Sexting%20Typology%20Bulletin_4-6-11_revised.pdf

References

18 U.S.C. §2252B.
18 U.S.C. §2252C.
18 U.S.C. §2256.
American Counseling Association. (2014). *ACA code of ethics*. Alexandria, VA: Author.
Ashcroft v. Free Speech Coalition, 535 U.S. 234 (2002).

Behun, R. J., & Cerrito, J. A. (2016). Defining child abuse for professional counselors as mandated reporters in Pennsylvania under the newly amended Child Protective Services Law. *Journal of the Pennsylvania Counseling Association, 15*(1), 39–43. Retrieved from www.pacounseling.org/aws/PACA/asset_manager/get_file/129165?ver=122

Behun, R. J., Cerrito, J. A., Delmonico, D. L., & Campenni, C. E. (2017). Curricular abstinence: Examining human sexuality training in school counselor preparation programs. *Journal of School Counseling, 15*(14). Retrieved from www.jsc.montana.edu/articles/v15n14.pdf

Behun, R. J., Cerrito, J. A., Delmonico, D. L., & Kolbert, J. (2019). The influence of personal and professional characteristics on school counselors' recognition and reporting of child sexual abuse. *Journal of School Counseling, 17*(13). Retrieved from www.jsc.montana.edu/articles/v17n13.pdf

Behun, R. J., Owens, E. W., & Cerrito, J. A. (2015). The amended Child Protective Services Law: New requirements for professional counselors as mandated reporters in Pennsylvania. *Journal of the Pennsylvania Counseling Association, 14*(2), 79–85. Retrieved from www.pacounseling.org/aws/PACA/asset_manager/get_file/113401?ver=159

Behun, R. J., Sweeney, V., Delmonico, D. L., & Griffin, E. J. (2012). Filtering and monitoring Internet content: A primer for helping professionals. *Sexual Addiction and Compulsivity, 19*, 140–155. doi: 10.1080/10720162.2012.666425

Child Protection and Obscenity Act of 1988, Pub. L. No. 100-690, 102 Stat. 4181, 4485–89, codified as amended at 18 U.S.C. § 2257.

Criminal Code, R.S.C., 1985, c. C-46. Retrieved from https://laws-lois.justice.gc.ca/eng/acts/C-46/page-37.html#h-118363

Digital Economy Act of 2017, c. 30. Retrieved from www.legislation.gov.uk/ukpga/2017/30/contents/enacted/data.htm

FindLaw. (2019). *State revenge porn laws*. Retrieved from https://criminal.findlaw.com/criminal-charges/revenge-porn-laws-by-state.html

Herlihy, B., & Corey, G. (2015). *ACA ethical standards casebook* (7th ed.). Alexandria, VA: ACA.

Miller v. California, 413 U.S. 15 (1973).

New York v. Ferber, 458 U.S. 747 (1982).

Obscene Publications Act of 1959, c. 66. Retrieved from www.legislation.gov.uk/ukpga/Eliz2/7-8/66/contents

Slane, A. (2013). Sexting and the law in Canada. *Canadian Journal of Human Sexuality, 22*(3), 117–122. doi:10.3138/cjhs.22.3.C01

Wolak, J., & Finkelhor, D. (2011, March). Sexting: A typology. *Crimes Against Children Research Center Bulletin*. Retrieved from www.unh.edu/ccrc/pdf/CV231_Sexting%20Typology%20Bulletin_4-6-11_revised.pdf

8 What's new? Current issues in youth and internet pornography

> I've been in this field for a long time. I try to keep up with everything that's going on, but it can be hard, you know? Technology is one of those things . . . you can never keep up, but I guess you can try. I saw this video the other day. It was of a politician running for national office. She was saying these crazy things that are totally opposite of her political platform. It was sent to me by a friend who has a different political point of view with the caption, "See, I told you she's crazy." And I believed him, until someone told me it was a fake. So then I started reading about how easy it is to fake videos. I mean, I know all about Photoshop and airbrushing and all of that, but a video? That looks real? I started thinking about my clients and their privacy. I started thinking about myself and MY privacy. It's scary, you know?

As this quote from a helping professional explains, technology and SEIM are ever-evolving issues. Writing a book such as this one is a challenge for a number of reasons, one of which is that as soon as you complete research on a topic and write about it, there is new research to read, new topics to explore, and new issues at the forefront of technology and pornography.

The goal of this chapter is to review some of the most pertinent emerging issues related to technology and SEIM. Because technology evolves so quickly, encapsulating all the current issues in the field can be nearly impossible. However, there are several specific areas that should be of concern to helping professionals working with adolescents who consume SEIM. In this chapter, we highlight three issues that have taken on specific prominence recently. First, we explore how societies, and specifically governments, are addressing issues related to SEIM and its consumption by adolescents. Second, we examine the development of *deepfake* technology, the artificial intelligence (AI) processes that allow people to create nearly undetectable fake images and videos, including the superimposing of others' faces on the bodies of those actors and actresses found in SEIM. Finally, we discuss the issue of sexting or sending provocative or explicit images using technology or posting them online.

After reading this chapter, you should be able to

1   Understand the challenges inherent in attempting to legislate SEIM, especially as those efforts relate to free speech rights as well as the accuracy of the information used to create legislation;

2   Identify what deepfake technology is and how it can be used to create SEIM that can be harmful and embarrassing to others; and
3   Appreciate the various means in which adolescents may engage in sexting, as well as the inherent risks associated with the practice.

Protected speech or protecting the public: government involvement in SEIM

For as long as there has been pornography, there have been challenges to pornography. Many of these challenges are made on the basis of moral or religious grounds. However, laws related to free or protected speech have often been used as a means of protecting an individual's right to view, or produce, pornography. This continued debate "spans a continuum between individual rights on one extreme and complete restriction of such material for society's good on the other extreme" (Perrin et al., 2008, p. 11). If we consider the argument that pornography is a societal issue that should be regulated by government entities, we should consider the potential harm that may come from the consumption of SEIM and other forms of pornography (Perrin et al., 2008). If we believe that pornography is harmful, then it can logically follow that our elected leaders have a responsibility to protect the public from that harm. That protection can come in the form of legislation that limits, or even outright bans, the production or consumption of pornography. Similar arguments have been used regarding the production and consumption of alcohol (e.g., U.S. prohibition laws) and illegal drugs (e.g., prohibitions on marijuana, opiates), and even the requirement in some jurisdictions that motorcycle riders wear protective helmets.

However, if we consider the consumption of pornography as an individual right, then the responsibility for using that right responsibly falls to the individual, or in the case of minors, that individual's legal guardians (Perrin et al., 2008). When we examine the issue through this lens, the issue becomes an exercise in free speech and individual choice, and the right to produce and consume pornography becomes protected in many societies. As Justice Thurgood Marshall of the U.S. Supreme Court wrote in the case of Stanley v Georgia (1969), "If the First Amendment means anything, it means that a State has no business telling a man sitting in his own house what books he may read or what films he may watch" (p. 565). While these rights are not absolute, such as in the case of possession of child pornography, Justice Marshall did make the case that pornography and free speech cannot be separated.

In the United States, federal legislation aimed at limiting adolescent access to SEIM and pornography has been enacted, only to later be overturned by federal courts. In 1996, Congress passed the Communication Decency Act (CDA) that was designed to limit access to SEIM for anyone under 18 years of age. The law was challenged in federal court on the basis of free speech and First Amendment protections. In the landmark case, Reno v. ACLU (1997), the U.S. Supreme Court struck down the CDA as unconstitutional because it might infringe upon the free speech rights of adults. In 2000, the Children's Internet Protection Act (CIPA) was enacted that limited funding to public places, such as schools and libraries, unless those entities incorporated software to limit inline access to SEIM by minors. Eventually, the law was challenged, but the U.S. Supreme Court found the CIPA constitutional (United States v. American Libraries Association, 2003).

While the argument related to free speech in the United States is largely based on the First Amendment of the U.S. Constitution, the protection of speech is not limited to one nation. Article 19 of the Universal Declaration on Human Rights states, "Everyone has the right to freedom of expression; this right includes freedom . . . to seek, receive, and impart information and ideas through any media and regardless of frontiers" (United Nations, 2015, p. 40). Similarly, Article 10 of the European Convention on Human Rights (ECHR) states, "Everyone has the right to freedom of expression. This right shall include the freedom to hold opinions and to receive and impart information and ideas without interference by public authority" (ECHR, 2010, p. 11). Governments pass their own laws that may or may not protect individual speech and expression; it is important for helping professionals to understand the statutes that govern pornography in their own jurisdictions.

For example, in the European Union, legislation was passed that would require ISPs to treat all online traffic equally and without discrimination, effectively supporting the concept of *net neutrality* (Buchanan, 2015). Net neutrality refers to the idea that all Internet traffic is treated equally, regardless of content. The legislation makes it difficult to enact laws that would create SEIM filters online, especially "opt-in" filters that would be required in order to view SEIM. Net neutrality has long been a contentious issue for governments, consumers, and companies that offer access to the Internet. Often identified as a free speech issue, challenges to net neutrality are perceived as limits on the access to information outlined by the U.S. Constitution, the United Nations, and the ECHR.

However, in the United Kingdom., the Digital Economy Act was recently passed that requires an Internet user to verify her or his age prior to accessing SEIM. As this chapter is being written, enactment of these provisions of the Digital Economy Act has been delayed due to administrative concerns (Burgess, 2019). While the stated purpose of the legislation is to limit access to SEIM to those over the age of 18, opponents of the law have argued that the security of users' information may be at risk and individual privacy could be jeopardized. Enforcement of the provisions would be the responsibility of the owner of the website, which would require tracking user's access to each site to ensure compliance with the law. Any verification system would have access to every SEIM site that a user has accessed. These data are obvious sensitive and private, and any breach could have significant consequences to user privacy.

Recent governmental efforts in the United States have examined the issue of pornography as a public health crisis; however, this movement started several decades earlier. In the 1980s, then U.S. Surgeon General, C. Everett Koop enlisted a panel of researchers and clinicians to examine the issue of pornography as a public health issue. The results of their work concluded that pornography does lead to attitudes, beliefs, and behaviors that have significant consequences for individuals and for society, and that the outcomes impair the emotional and physical health of both children and adults (Koop, 1987). Since the release of the report, the issue of public health and pornography has been hotly contested.

Almost three decades later, an organization called the National Center on Sexual Exploitation (NCSE) hosted a symposium in Washington, DC, called *Pornography: A Public Health Crisis* (NCSE, 2015). During this event, a number of speakers presented papers on research in the field of pornography, SEIM, and adolescents. Among the topics discussed were the relationships between explicit material and violence against women and children, issues related to adolescent brain development, and concerns about pornography and human trafficking (NCSE, 2015). In one of the presentations at the symposium, Ernie Allen argued that a host of factors have contributed to the emergence of pornography as a public health crisis, including ubiquitous access to the Internet, a lack of effective legislation, lack of prosecution, and a failure in educating parents about the concerns raised by the NCSE (Allen, 2015).

The executive summary of the report published by the NCSE states that the purpose of the symposium and its supporting documents

> is to bring together Members of Congress, their staffs, the national press, and the public to educate on the public health crisis resulting from pornography and sexual exploitation. . . . This briefing is intended to demonstrate that pornography has caused a public health crisis and we hope Congress receives this message and responds accordingly.
>
> (Hawkins, 2015, p. 4)

While the U.S. Congress has not taken any significant action since the symposium, individual states have. As the time of publication, 16 states have passed some form of resolution recognizing pornography as a public health issue (Fight the New Drug, 2019). Those states include Arkansas (House Resolution), Arizona (House Resolution), Florida (House Resolution), Florida (House Resolution), Idaho (House Concurring Resolution), Kansas (House Resolution), Kentucky (Senate Resolution), Louisiana (House Resolution), Missouri (Senate Concurring Resolution), Montana (House Resolution), Oklahoma (House Concurring Resolution), Pennsylvania (House Resolution), South Dakota (Senate Concurring Resolution), Tennessee (Senate Joint Resolution), Utah (Senate Concurring Resolution), Utah (Senate Concurring Resolution), and Virginia (House Resolution). These resolutions were passed between 2016, with Utah being the first to do so, and 2019, when Montana passed the *Resolution on the Public Health Crisis of Pornography*. It is important to note that resolutions hold no legal authority; they are not laws and do not require any action or prohibit any behavior. However, such resolutions can be used as the basis for other governmental actions such as decisions about funding or administrative policies.

The Utah resolution was a direct result of the 2015 NCSE Symposium aimed at federal lawmakers. During the summit, a Utah lawmaker named Todd Weiler took note and championed the resolution that was passed in his home state (Hamblin, 2016). That resolution makes statements that tie pornography consumption to violence and rape against women and children, abnormal brain development, biological addiction, a decrease in young male's desire to marry, dissatisfaction in marriage, and infidelity (Concurrent Resolution on the Public Health Crisis, 2016). Weiler claims that the resolution mirrored the statements presented at the NCSE gathering in Washington, DC, a year earlier.

However, the statements made in the Utah resolution, as well as those made at the NCSE meeting, have been refuted in the research. For example, the argument that pornography consumption leads to an increase in acts of rape has been refuted as early as 1991. Kutchinsky (1991) studied this issue examining the incidence of rape in four countries: Denmark, Sweden, Germany, and the United States because pornography was widely available in each of those countries at the time. The study found that the data on rape and other sexual offenses did not support the argument that pornography has detrimental effects as those effects relate to sexual violence (Kutchinsky, 1991).

Another statement made in the Utah resolution is that pornography has biologically addictive qualities and is as addictive as illegal drugs. However, those arguments have been challenged and refuted in scientific studies, as well. Prause, Steele, Staley, Sabatinelli, and Hajcak (2015) examined the electrical patterns in the brains of subjects who reported significant concerns with the consumption of sexually explicit material. In this study, those who reported difficulty modulating their use of pornography reported higher sexual desire as well as different brain functioning found in substance abuse models (Prause et al., 2015). In short, the study found that there was no support for a model of pornography addiction based on brain activity. Research also indicated that watching pornography did not negatively impact love but rather increased the desire for sex with a committed partner (Prause et al., 2015).

As authors of this text, we do not think it is our role to tell the reader what to think about these issues. Instead, we hope you will consider the various perspectives, viewpoints, and research studies and make an informed decision for yourself, based on facts, data, and, of course, your own moral compass. However, what we challenge the reader to consider is how much influence one's own morality should have on the development of a professional opinion. As helping professionals, we are responsible for bracketing our own beliefs so as not to allow those values to impact our work with clients. As discussed elsewhere in this text, as professionals we have an ethical obligation to prevent our own values from negatively impacting our work with clients.

The challenge inherent in this process lies in the conflicting data and various perspectives on SEIM, especially as it relates to adolescents. We can engage in confirmation bias quite easily; that is, we can focus on only the information that confirms our preconceived opinions and values and then use those data to support our opinions as facts. The research on adolescents and SEIM is full of contradictions and limitations that can allow us the opportunity to confirm our biases. However, the challenge we issue to the reader is instead to explore data and information that actively *challenges* your own opinions, values, and biases. Allow yourself to be challenged to see the issue "from the other side," so to speak, and give yourself the opportunity to develop a well-reasoned and informed opinion about these issues. Learning Activity 8.1 invites the reader to do just that.

Learning Activity 8.1

Seeing things from another point of view

One of the greatest challenges in our helping work is to separate our values and beliefs from our work with clients. One of the challenges inherent in this process is the effect of *confirmation bias*, which is when we focus our attention and memory on information that supports our previous viewpoints, often at the expense of data that may contradict those views.

We challenge the reader to consider the following statement: adolescent consumption of SEIM will lead to negative outcomes, such as sexual aggression.

As you read that statement, consider your initial response to it. Do you agree with the statement or not?

For this exercise, we suggest you work with a partner who has a different reaction to the statement. For example, if you agree that adolescent consumption of SEIM leads to sexual aggression, then find a partner who disagrees. Once you have found someone with whom to work, we suggest the following.

Take the opposing viewpoint. Have your partner do the same. Prepare to discuss this statement with your partner, which each of you engaging from the opposite point of view of the one you would normally hold.

Challenge yourself to investigate the opposite perspective. Look through the research literature. Examine different sources of information. Take some time to truly investigate the topic but from a perspective different from the one you normally hold. When you feel prepared, engage your partner in a respectful debate of the question. Hold firm to the perspective you're asked to maintain in this exercise. After you've finished your discussion, consider the following questions:

1. What did you learn about the topic of sexual aggression and adolescent consumption of SEIM that you may not have known before?
2. Did you find it difficult to debate a perspective different from your own? If so, what made that difficult? If it was easier than you expected, what contributed to that experience?
3. How did your partner react to your debating their point of view?
4. What, if anything, did this exercise teach you about confirmation bias?

Deepfakes: artificial intelligence and pornography

The term *deepfake* refers to videos or images that appear online that use sophisticated technology to graft one face on to another body (Weissman, 2018). In the case of images, these have been prevalent online for quite some time and can be made with a host of editing tools, such as Adobe Photoshop. However, in the case of deepfake videos, the process is completed through the use of sophisticated AI software that creates computer-generated models that can create videos that look quite real (Gallagher, 2018).

Deepfake videos have received a great deal of attention for their use in political campaigns and other popular culture (Parkin, 2019). For example, a 2019 video circulated online in which it appeared that Nancy Pelosi, Speaker of the U.S. House of Representatives, was intoxicated and slurring her words through a press conference. Donald Trump gave the video significant attention on Twitter. However, it was not a real video; it was created using deepfake technology. Another 2019 video of Facebook founder Mark Zuckerberg was doctored to make it appear that he was discussing the use of stolen user data for nefarious means. Zuckerberg never made such comments (Parkin, 2019).

Deepfake technology uses AI logarithms in order to match faces, expressions, and voice patterns of one subject to a video of a second subject. The technology was originally developed by a team led by Ian Goodfellow, a computer scientist who has worked at Google, among other companies. In 2014, Goodfellow and colleagues developed what is a relatively simple idea, two separate computer AI processes work against one another in order to continuously improve on the process until a relatively sophisticated result emerges. The process takes photographs of one subject, sometimes using hundreds or thousands of images, to match facial expressions, sometimes at a rate of 60 times per second (Goodfellow et al., 2014). Many of the tools to create deepfakes are available in Google's AI library and are free and available to the public.

As this technology developed, so did its use to create SEIM. For example, images of the actress Scarlett Johansson have been used to create a number of deepfake pornographic videos, one of which had been viewed over 1.5 million times on a popular SEIM site by the end of 2018 (Harwell, 2018). Images of celebrities are readily available across the Internet, making it relatively easy for those who have the technological know-how to create deepfake pornography. Johansson has called the practice "demeaning" but also believes that doing anything to prevent the creation of these videos or their distribution is a "lost cause" (Kelly, 2019, para. 2). Similar deepfake pornographic videos have been created with images of musician Taylor Swift, former U.S. first lady Michelle Obama, and British duchesses Meghan Markle and Kate Middleton (Gallagher, 2018).

However, as the technology becomes more advanced and images of everyday people are easier to obtain through social media sites, such as Instagram, deepfake pornography has begun to impact those who do not hold celebrity status. Harwell (2018) describes the creation of a sexually explicit deepfake video made of a female in her 40s. The person who had the video made did not have the requisite technical knowledge to complete the task; he went to the Internet and found someone to do it for about US$20 (Harwell, 2018). The requester provided 491 images, many taken from the female's Facebook account, to the video's creator. The video was produced and delivered two days later. At the end of 2018, it had been viewed over 400 times.

Victims of deepfake pornography have little legal recourse, especially given how new the technology is and how quickly it has evolved. In the United Kingdom, producers of deepfake pornography can be prosecuted for harassment. In May 2018, a 25-year-old man was charged and convicted of harassment for using Photoshop to create deepfake images of an intern at his place of employment and posting them to SEIM sites online (Nelson, 2018). The man was sentenced to spend 16 weeks in prison and ordered to pay a fine of £5,000.

However, such prosecutions are not always easy or even possible according to some legal experts. In the United States, for example, deepfake images and videos may be protected as free speech under the First Amendment of the Constitution. Specifically, deepfakes may be considered parodies or satire, which have traditionally been protected as free speech (Ellis, 2018). If a deepfake is built using public images, the deepfake video or image may be protected as a new artistic creation (Harwell, 2018). However, the Electronic Frontier Foundation has argued that there may be both criminal and civil remedies for individuals who are victims of deepfake pornography (Greene, 2018). For example, if the creator of the deepfake SEIM were to pressure someone to pay to have the video removed from an Internet site, extortion laws might be applicable. Also, laws related to harassment might be used criminally, like in the aforementioned case in the United Kingdom.

One civil remedy a deepfake victim may have in the United States is under the *false light* invasion of privacy statutes (Greene, 2018). Recognized in about two-thirds of the United States, false light statutes commonly address photo distortions, manipulations, and embellishments. In order to win a false light lawsuit, the victim of the deepfake must prove that he or she was harmed in some way – for example, that his or her reputation was damaged or the person suffered emotional pain or anguish (Greene, 2018). Defamation laws may also be applicable in deepfake cases as well as copyright infringement in cases where an image used in the deepfake process was copyrighted.

Another legal recourse that a victim of deepfakes may have is through the *revenge porn* laws that exist throughout the United States to include 41 states and the District of Columbia (FindLaw, 2019). Revenge porn is considered a form of harassment in which sexually explicit images are distributed online without the consent of the person whose image is being distributed. Despite the term revenge porn, revenge does not have to be the purpose of the distribution; in many states, the victim need only prove that the image or video distributed without their consent and was meant to annoy or harass the victim (FindLaw, 2019).

However, the law is still unclear, and until more cases are brought and the courts create more precedent, it is uncertain what legal recourse victims of deepfakes may have. In addition to the ambiguity in the law, it can be very difficult to trace a deepfake to its creator. Several organizations are working to eliminate deepfakes from online platforms. For example, Google has included deepfake products in its ban list, allowing users to request the search engine block results that display deepfakes (Harwell, 2018). The online platform Reddit has banned deepfakes from its site, as has the SEIM site Pornhub (Gallagher, 2018). However, these efforts have done little to stem the deepfake tide.

Sexting: "send nudes"

The phrase "send nudes" has become part of the adolescent lexicon that represents the notion of sexting. *Sexting* is the process of taking sexual images of oneself and then sharing those images with others; it is the act of sharing digital images of oneself with someone else, usually for purposes such as sexual arousal, flirting, or expressing romantic interest in someone. It is estimated that as many as 60% of adolescents have engaged in sexting, depending on how the term is defined (Peter & Valkenburg, 2016).

When we consider sexting, the definition provided at the opening of this section may prove useful, but in reality, sexting is much more complex. For example, sexting may include the act of creating and sending sexually explicit images of oneself; it may also include the act of requesting or receiving those images (Temple & Choi, 2014). Another issue related to sexting is the forwarding of an image to someone other than the intended recipient (Lippman & Campbell, 2014). Another consideration when we try to define sexting is the content of the image – that is, what sexual characteristics must be present in order for an image to be considered sexting? The definitions vary across the research, from depictions of sexual acts to partially nude images or images of someone clothed but in a sexual or provocative pose (Barrense-Dias, Berchtold, Suris, & Arke, 2017).

Another consideration of sexting is how the image is transmitted. While much sexting behavior occurs between two people using smartphones, tablets, or computers, another method is the posting of images on social media sites (i.e., Snapchat, Twitter) or other Internet sites. This also raises issues related to *revenge porn*, which was discussed previously in this chapter. While sexting is generally considered a consensual act between two people, the term revenge porn is generally viewed as a nonconsensual act. For example, someone may send a partner a sexual image of him or herself, assuming that the image will not be distributed. The recipient of the image (or even someone else to whom the image was later forwarded) might post that image online. As discussed previously, civil and criminal statutes can be used to hold people accountable for engaging in acts of revenge porn, but it can be difficult to prosecute.

While sexting is often considered harmless among adolescents, the research literature is mixed on this assumption (Gómez & Ayala, 2014; Ricketts, Maloney, Marcum, & Higgins, 2015). While sexting has been discussed in the research as a consensual practice between two people for the purpose of expressing romantic interest (Crimmins & Seigfried-Spellar, 2014), the act of sexting may also have a number of potential negative effects. Sexting can lead to harassment, humiliation, and bullying (O'Sullivan, 2014; Crimmins & Seigfried-Spellar, 2014). Additionally, the act of sending or receiving explicit images of minors might be prosecuted under child pornography statutes (Ricketts et al., 2015).

As practitioners in the helping professions, it is vital that we are aware of the ways adolescents engage with one another online, including the act of sexting. While it may be considered harmless flirting or something that "everyone does," the consequences can be significant. Once an image is shared, it cannot be taken back. The person who possesses the image may choose to share it, and even if it is shared with only one person, that person may share it with others. One image sent consensually from one teenager to another can make its way across the Internet with lightning speed and removing an image that has "gone viral" is virtually impossible. While there may be civil or criminal remedies for a victim of such behavior, the humiliation and embarrassment are not so easily resolved.

Psychoeducation is critical when working with adolescents and the topic of sexting. While the phrase "send nudes" may be ubiquitous among this population, the behavior need not be. If we work to make our clients aware of the potential dangers of sexting, we may be able to help inform decision-making and impact behavior.

While someone may want to impress a potential partner with nude selfies, the result may not be what one hopes for. Prevention is critical and psychoeducation for both senders and receivers of sexting images is paramount. Learning Activity 8.2 invites the reader to consider a case study related to this topic.

Learning Activity 8.2

I never thought it would go this far

As we consider issues related to sexting, read the following case illustration and then consider the questions that follow:

David is a 15-year-old male who you've been working with for about a year. You and David have developed a good rapport, and he has been honest with you about a relationship he has developed with another boy in his school. David identifies as gay, and he has come out to his parents, classmates, and teachers. David has been developing a relationship with another boy named Chris, who is still exploring his sexuality and has identified as questioning.

David and Chris have been flirting on and off for several weeks, and their relationship has become physical, but without any sexual intercourse. David has had one previous sexual encounter with another boy his age; Chris has had several sexual experiences but exclusively with girls his own age or older. This is the first time Chris has engaged in a physical relationship with another male.

One night when Chris and David were texting, David asked Chris if he would send him a nude image of his genitals. David tells you that at first, Chris was hesitant, but then he agreed on the condition that David would delete the photo at the end of their text chat and would never share it with anyone. "I was absolutely going to delete it," David tells you, "but to be honest, it was a turn on, and I wanted to keep it so I could get turned on anytime I looked at it."

David explains that he and Chris got into an argument when Chris expressed his attraction to a girl in their class. The argument became so intense that David told Chris that he didn't want to see him anymore and that their relationship was over. That night, David was very upset and decided to try to get revenge on Chris by sending the nude image to the girl Chris had expressed attraction for with the message, "Chris wants you so you can have this." That girl then forwarded the image to about 10 classmates in a group chat, describing who the image was and how she received it.

"I really can't believe this," David says. "It was just a fight, and I was just mad. I can't believe this happened. What am I going to do?"

Questions for consideration:

1 What are the main elements in this case? What are the different issues to which you should be attending?

2   Are there any legal or ethical issues for you to consider as a helping professional? (This question may require you to research your professional code of ethics and legal issues in your jurisdiction.)
3   As a helping professional, is there anything you could have done to prevent this from happening? How would you have implemented those interventions?
4   How do you answer David's question, "What am I going to do?"

Conclusion

This chapter explored three issues that are prominent in the study of adolescents and the consumption of SEIM. A discussion of the intersection of society and SEIM examined various legislative actions that have attempted to prevent adolescent access to SEIM, as well as how governments have addressed SEIM, in general. This chapter also examined issues related to deepfake technology, the process of using evolving technology to superimpose a face on to different sexual image or video for the purpose of creating a lifelike image of that person engaged in SEIM. Finally, we discussed the issue of sexting, or engaging in sharing explicit photos or images of oneself with others, either directly or through Internet websites and social media platforms. Throughout this chapter, the goal was to challenge helping practitioners to consider how they can best intervene with adolescent consumers of SEIM, as that consumption relates to each of these topics.

Summary

- Laws related to free or protected speech have often been used as a means of protecting an individual's right to view, or produce, pornography.
- The debate over regulating SEIM is typically a struggle between two opposing perspectives. One perspective is that SEIM is a form of free speech, protected by laws such as the First Amendment of the U.S. Constitution. An alternative perspective is that SEIM poses a public health issue that must be addressed for the good of society at large.
- Laws have been passed in the United States and elsewhere that have attempted to limit access to pornography and SEIM, many of which have been overturned by the courts.
- The argument as to whether pornography and SEIM are a public health crisis is based largely on research that has been challenged by studies that have produced disparate results.
- The term *deepfake* refers to videos or images that appear online that use sophisticated technology to graft one face on to another body. Deepfake technology uses AI logarithms in order to match faces, expressions, and voice patterns of one subject to a video of a second subject.

- As deepfake technology developed, so too did its use to create SEIM, including deepfake images and videos featuring the faces of popular culture icons superimposed on pornographic actors and actresses.
- As technology becomes more advanced and images of everyday people are easier to obtain through social media sites, deepfake pornography has begun to impact those who do not hold celebrity status. A deepfake video can be created for as little as $20 and requires only a few hundred images of the victim.
- While there are legal remedies for victims of deepfake videos and images, prosecution is difficult, if not sometimes impossible.
- *Sexting* can be defined as the process of using a phone, computer, or tablet to take sexual images of oneself and then sending those images to others. However, sexting may also include the posting of images or videos to social media sites or other Internet locations.
- While sexting has been discussed in the research as a consensual practice between two people for the purpose of expressing romantic interest, the act of sexting also has a number of potential negative effects such as embarrassment or harassment.
- Sexting can also be used to produce revenge porn, which is when images or videos are circulated online without the consent of the individual pictured. There is legal recourse for victims of revenge porn, but like deepfakes, prosecution can be difficult.

Additional resources

In print

Gómez, L. C., & Ayala, E. S. (2014). Psychological aspects, attitudes and behaviour related to the practice of sexting: A systematic review of the existent literature. *Procedia–Social and Behavioral Sciences*, *132*, 114–120. doi:10.1016/j.sbspro.2014.04.286

National Center on Sexual Exploitation. (2015). *Pornography: A public health crisis*. Washington, DC: Author.

On the web

Harwell, D. (2018, December 30). Fake-porn videos are being weaponized to harass and humiliate women: "Everybody is a potential target." *The Washington Post*. Retrieved from www.washingtonpost.com/technology/2018/12/30/fake-porn-videos-are-being-weaponized-harass-humiliate-women-everybody-is-potential-target/?utm_term=.742c0a413708

National Center on Sexual Exploitation. (2015). *Pornography: A public health crisis*. Retrieved from http://endsexualexploitation.org/wp-content/uploads/NCOSE_SymposiumBriefingBooklet_9-2_final_web.pdf

References

Allen, E. (2015). Why is finding a solution so difficult? In National Center on Sexual Exploitation (Ed.), *Pornography: A public health crisis*. Retrieved from http://

endsexualexploitation.org/wp-content/uploads/NCOSE_SymposiumBriefingBooklet_9-2_final_web.pdf

Barrense-Dias, Y., Berchtold, A., Suris, J., & Arke, C. (2017). Sexting and the definition issue. *Journal of Adolescent Health, 61*, 544–554. doi:10.1016/j.jadohealth.2017.05.009

Buchanan, R. T. (2015, October 28). E.U. rules U.K.'s "porn filters" are illegal. *The Independent*. Retrieved from www.independent.co.uk/life-style/gadgets-and-tech/news/eu-rules-uks-porn-filters-are-illegal-a6711756.html

Burgess, M. (2019, June 20). This is how age verification will work under the U.K.'s porn law. *Wired*. Retrieved from www.wired.co.uk/article/uk-porn-age-verification

Crimmins, D. M., & Seigfried-Spellar, K. C. (2014). Peer attachment, sexual experiences, and risky online behaviors as predictors of sexting behaviors among undergraduate students. *Computers in Human Behavior, 32*, 268–275. doi:10.1016/j.chb.2013.12.012

Ellis, E. G. (2018, January 26). People can put your face on porn-and the law can't help you. *Wired*. Retrieved from www.wired.com/story/face-swap-porn-legal-limbo/

European Convention on Human Rights. (2010). *The convention for the protection of human rights and fundamental freedoms*. Retrieved from www.echr.coe.int/Documents/Convention_ENG.pdf

Fight the New Drug. (2019). *These 16 states passed resolutions recognizing porn as a public health issue*. Retrieved from https://fightthenewdrug.org/here-are-the-states-that-have-passed-resolutions/

FindLaw. (2019). *State revenge porn laws*. Retrieved from https://criminal.findlaw.com/criminal-charges/revenge-porn-laws-by-state.html

Gallagher, S. (2018, November 21). What is deepfake pornography and is it illegal in the U.K.? *Huffington Post*. Retrieved from www.huffingtonpost.co.uk/entry/what-is-deep-fake-pornography-and-is-it-illegal-in-the-uk

Gómez, L. C., & Ayala, E. S. (2014). Psychological aspects, attitudes and behaviour related to the practice of sexting: A systematic review of the existent literature. *Procedia–Social and Behavioral Sciences, 132*, 114–120. doi:10.1016/j.sbspro.2014.04.286

Goodfellow, I. J., Pouget-Abadie, J., Mirza, M., Xu, B., Warde-Farley, D., Ozair, S., . . . Yoshua, B. (2014, December). *Generative adversarial nets*. Poster session presented at the annual convention on Neural Information Processing Systems. Montreal, Canada.

Greene, D. (2018, February 13). We don't need new laws for faked videos, we already have them. *Electronic Frontier Foundation*. Retrieved from www.eff.org/deeplinks/2018/02/we-dont-need-new-laws-faked-videos-we-already-have-them

Hamblin, J. (2016, April 14). Inside the movement to declare pornography a "health crisis." *The Atlantic*. Retrieved from www.theatlantic.com/health/archive/2016/04/a-crisis-of-education/478206/

Harwell, D. (2018, December 30). Fake-porn videos are being weaponized to harass and humiliate women: "Everybody is a potential target." *The Washington Post*. Retrieved from www.washingtonpost.com/technology/2018/12/30/fake-porn-videos-are-being-weaponized-harass-humiliate-women-everybody-is-potential-target/?utm_term=.742c0a413708

Hawkins, D. (2015). Executive summary. In National Center on Sexual Exploitation (Ed.), *Pornography: A public health crisis*. Retrieved from http://endsexualexploitation.org/wp-content/uploads/NCOSE_SymposiumBriefingBooklet_9-2_final_web.pdf

Kelly, E. (2019, January 2). Scarlett Johansson says there's nothing that can stop people using her in "deepfake" porn. *Metro*. Retrieved from https://metro.co.uk/2019/01/02/scarlett-johansson-says-nothing-can-stop-people-using-deepfake-porn-8300841/

Koop, C. E. (1987). Report of the Surgeon General's workshop on pornography and public health. *American Psychologist, 42*(10), 944–945. doi:10.1037/0003-066X.42.10.944

Kutchinsky, B. (1991). Pornography and rape: Theory and practice? Evidence from crime data in four countries where pornography is easily available. *International Journal of Law and Psychiatry, 14*(1–2), 47–64. doi:10.1016/0160-2527(91)90024-H

Lippman, J. R., & Campbell, S. W. (2014). Damned if you do, damned if you don't . . . If you're a girl: Relational and normative contexts of adolescent sexting in the United States. *Journal of Children and Media, 8*, 371–386. doi:10.1080/17482798.2014.923009

National Center on Sexual Exploitation. (2015). *Pornography: A public health crisis*. Retrieved from http://endsexualexploitation.org/wp-content/uploads/NCOSE_SymposiumBriefingBooklet_9-2_final_web.pdf

Nelson, S. C. (2018, June 24). "Deepfake porn" and "cyber-flashing": The other abuses not included in new upskirting laws. *Huffington Post*. Retrieved from www.huffingtonpost.co.uk/entry/upskirting-bill-should-cover-deepfake-porn-and-cyber-flashing-too_uk_5b2b9e70e4b0321a01ce6ed8

O'Sullivan, L. (2014). Linking online sexual activities to health outcomes among teens. *New Directions for Child and Adolescent Development, 2014*(144), 37–51. doi:10.1002/cad.20059

Parkin, S. (2019, June 22). Politicians fear this like fire: The rise of the deepfake and the threat to democracy. *The Guardian*. Retrieved from www.theguardian.com/technology/ng-interactive/2019/jun/22/the-rise-of-the-deepfake-and-the-threat-to-democracy

Perrin, P. C., Madanat, H. N., Barnes, M. D., Carolan, A., Clark, R. B., Ivins, N., . . . Williams, P. N. (2008). Health education's role in framing pornography as a public health issue: Local and national strategies with international implications. *Global Health Promotion, 15*, 11–18. doi:10.1177/1025382307088093

Peter, J., & Valkenburg, P. M. (2016). Adolescents and pornography: A review of 20 years of research. *The Journal of Sex Research, 53*(4–5), 509–531. doi: 10.1080/00224499.2016.1143441

Prause, N., Steele, V. R., Staley, C., Sabatinelli, D., & Hajcak, G. (2015). Modulation of late positive potentials by sexual images in problem users and controls inconsistent with "porn addiction." *Biological Psychology, 109*, 192–199. doi:10.1016/j.biopsycho.2015.06.005

Reno v. ACLU, 521 U.S. 844 (1997).

Ricketts, M., Maloney, L., Marcum, C., & Higgins, C. (2015). The effect of Internet related problems on the sexting behaviors of juveniles. *American Journal of Criminal Justice, 40*(2), 270–284. doi:10.1007/s12103-014-9247-5

Stanley v. Georgia, 394 U.S. 557 (1969).

Temple, J. R., & Choi, H. (2014). Longitudinal association between teen sexting and sexual behavior. *Pediatrics, 134*(5), E1287–E1292. doi:10.1542/peds.2014-1974

United Nations. (2015). *Universal declaration of human rights*. Retrieved from www.un.org/en/udhrbook/pdf/udhr_booklet_en_web.pdf

United States v. American Libraries Association, 2539 U.S. 194. (2003).

Weissman, C. G. (2018, February 13). Are deepfakes legal? Here's what the law says about the creepy video mashups. *Fast Company*. Retrieved from www.fastcompany.com/40530634/are-deepfakes-legal-heres-what-the-law-says-about-the-creepy-video-mashups

9 Conclusion

Making sense of it all

> There's so much to know. There's all of this research about kids and the Internet and how they use it to access pornography. But what does it all mean? How do I make sense of it all? What is important and what isn't? I work with kids every day, and they are always on their phones, on their tablets, on laptops. They're constantly online, and I can't imagine it's good for them. But is it all as bad as it seems from what I've been reading and learning about?

Maybe things do not "seem bad" to you or maybe they do. But the vignette here demonstrates the challenge inherent for helping professionals as they attempt to sift through all the data and information available about the impact of technology and pornography on young people.

Our purpose in this chapter is to help the reader to conceptualize what has come before. There are many studies in the research literature. There are miles of data through which to sift. While there are some suggestions in the literature about how best to address adolescent consumption of SEIM, there are no definite ideas or "magic bullets" to address concerns, if there are even concerns that should be addressed. Because the literature is mixed and causal research studies are almost nonexistent, one might make the argument that adolescent consumption of SEIM is not a problem, so no solution is necessary.

Each chapter of this text begins with a numbered list of outcomes we hope the reader will achieve after reading the book. This chapter is different. There is only one learning objective for this chapter of the text; our hope after reading this chapter is that you will have a better context for understanding and using what you have read to this point in order to help the young people with whom you work.

Technology as a cultural construct

Throughout this text, we discuss technology as a generational issue and, as such, a cultural construct. Prensky's (2001) seminal work on digital natives and digital immigrants provides the context for addressing this in our work as helping professionals, and Hoffman (2013) specifically examined how technology impacts the helping relationship and the development of a therapeutic alliance. Hoffman

(2013) makes an excellent argument that technology should be viewed as a cultural construct in relation to the helping process. If culture consists of elements such as how we communicate, how we perceive the world, and how we engage with others, then technology is certainly worth considering in discussions about culture.

The impact of technology on the relationship between people from different generations has long been a challenge. When we consider Generation Y and Millennials and their relationships with Generation X and Baby Boomers, we see the disconnect. It is what Prensky (2001) identified so clearly in his work regarding digital natives and digital immigrants. But for members of Generation X, they felt misunderstood by Baby Boomers, and technology was part of that divide. Music videos, video game systems, personal computers, and other technology that was "native" to Generation X was not understood by previous generations. For Baby Boomers, it was the conflict with the Greatest Generation over Elvis Presley on the television and the Beatles on the radio.

When it comes to how best to bridge these digital divides, we can find direction if we consider these differences as cultural, not just generational or technological. Cultural competence is developed through the development of our own knowledge, skill, and attitudes about cultures other than our own, as well as the people who identify when them (Ratts, Singh, Nassar-McMillan, Butler, & McCullough, 2016). If we look at those from other cultures as "wrong," we are bound to struggle in our connections. If we assume that the teenager who is staring at his or her phone is somehow disconnected from the world, we may be missing the fact that this young person is more connected to the world than previous generations ever were. Time spent on the phone may include texting with dozens of friends and peers or connecting on social media with people around the globe.

Helping professionals must challenge themselves to consider their own values, beliefs, and attitudes about technology and the young people who live in a digital world. When we consider knowledge, we can ask ourselves how much we know and understand technology. While we may not become Instagram famous, we might benefit from knowing what it is and how it works. How skilled are we at navigating a digital world, and can we grow from immigrants into this new technological era? Do we judge the teenager who is staring intently at their tablet screen, or can we take a moment to reflect on our own biases about technology and make efforts to correct our blind spots and empathize with our clients?

Attitudes, behaviors, and self-image

Chapters 3–5 discussed the relationships between adolescent consumption of SEIM and the development of attitudes, behaviors, and one's image of the self. While research findings vary widely, and there is certainly ambiguity about what it all might mean for the helping practitioner, what we can glean from the findings is that when it comes to interventions, education is key. Several studies (Perrin et al., 2008; Peter & Valkenburg, 2009; To, Kan, & Ngain, 2013; Tsitsika et al., 2009; Wallmyr & Welin, 2006) suggest that education is critical to addressing these issues. Certainly, if we have learned nothing else from the literature, we do know that education about sexuality is woefully inadequate in many communities and many adolescents do seek out information online about sexuality, relationships, and gender expectations.

If we know that education can be a critical factor in helping adolescents as they navigate the world of Internet pornography, then doing what we can to educate young people becomes a central focus of our work. Certainly, it is important for the helping professional to be as knowledgeable as possible about SEIM and the Internet; this is why the earlier chapters in the text are research oriented. But education about SEIM is more than simply reading a text or a few research articles. We do not necessarily have to consume SEIM ourselves, but we can also learn by asking questions of our clients, by reading information in other media, such as reliable news sources, and we can participate in continuing education around these issues.

It is also important to consider the specifics of how we focus our psychoeducational efforts. In many communities, we find inadequate education about sexuality, pornography, and online safety. But when we do provide sexual education, do we educate young people about SEIM? If we consider the benefits of providing a counterpoint to what adolescents see online and in other forms of media, perhaps we can challenge the messages found in SEIM and other media and mitigate the potential negative impact of these media. Peter and Valkenburg (2009) stress this point clearly in their research in this area.

It is also important that we not allow our own discomfort or our own biases to prevent us from being objective consumers of information. As helping professionals learn more about SEIM and its potential influence on young people, we should be aware of our own confirmation biases, our own value judgments, and our own choices when it comes to what we choose to learn. When we share our knowledge with clients, and as they share their stories with us, we should be open to honest, mature, two-way conversation. If a client presented to us and said, "I am having a problem because of my beliefs about religion," it might be challenging. We may not hold the same spiritual beliefs and that could make our work difficult, but ethical helping professionals find ways to bracket those personal reactions for the benefit of the client. It should be no different when a client presents and says, "I'm having a problem because of my beliefs about pornography."

The intersection of culture and pornography

As discussed in Chapter 6, there are a host of cultural influences that can impact young people's consumption of, and perception of SEIM and other forms of pornography. Research indicates that age and gender can be influences on SEIM use (Beggan & Allison, 2003; Bleakley, Hennessy, & Fishbein, 2011; Rasmussen & Bierman, 2016; Tsaliki, 2011). Political ideology (Häggström-Nordin, Sandberg, Hanson, & Tydén, 2006) and worldview (Perry & Schleifer, 2017) may also have influence. Religious beliefs are important to consider with regard to SEIM consumption (Perry, 2018) as is sexual identity (Træen, Nilsen, & Stigum, 2006).

But knowing that various cultural influences can relate to how, when, and to what extent young people consume SEIM is only part of the equation. What is also important is how helping professionals can use these data to support young people in their emotional and sexual development. Obviously, understanding these issues is imperative, but finding ways to use this knowledge in the helping relationship is key. As we consider culture generally, issues of knowledge, skill, and attitudes are central (Ratts et al., 2016). What is provided in Chapter 6 is the knowledge; however, developing skill in multicultural helping takes time and practice. Practicing our clinical skills and receiving appropriate supervision around issues of culture are imperative in our growth as helpers.

But what may be most important as we consider culture is the evolution of our personal values. Of course, we are not suggesting that one should change one's value system in order to work in the helping profession. However, we do often preach the virtues of meeting clients "where they are." That process includes empathy and the recognition of the value of others' beliefs. For example, religion can significantly impact SEIM consumption, as well as one's beliefs about SEIM use. As helpers, our beliefs are not the focus of the therapeutic relationship. Our religious beliefs may impart strong messages about pornography and sexuality. However, it is *our clients'* beliefs that are central to the helping process. This is true of the other topics discussed in Chapter 6, be it worldview, sexual identity, or politics. In fact, it is true of every cultural issue. Helpers should bracket their own beliefs and instead focus on the belief system of the client, without judgment or imposing their own values.

Ethics and the law

When working with minors in any context, understanding the law is critical, as is understanding our ethical responsibilities as helping professionals. When we consider issues related to sexuality and potential illegal activity, the importance of knowing our legal and ethical obligations become even more serious. There are many ethical and legal concerns related to sexuality, SEIM, and other forms of pornography that are specific to individuals under the age of legal consent (e.g., 18 years old in the United States). Having some cursory knowledge of these mandates can be crucial for our work.

As discussed in Chapter 7, understanding the differences between ethics and laws is important for successful work as a helping professional. For example, the ACA (2014) has its own Code of Ethics, which are based in the moral principles of autonomy, nonmaleficence, beneficence, justice, fidelity, and veracity. The Code of Ethics is complete with expectations of professional counselors and their work with clients, including minor clients. Some issues that are noteworthy include confidentiality, working within one's scope of competence, the bracketing of our own values, and research ethics when working with minors. Some of the critical legal issues for helping professionals include understanding the philosophical underpinnings of laws related to SEIM, mandated reporting, obscenity, child pornography, and legal issues around sexting.

A primer on academic research

Several chapters in this text focus heavily on the academic research related to youth consumption of Internet pornography. We included these studies because we believe it is important to be knowledgeable about the many relationships that have been explored by academic researchers across the world. These studies provide important context about topics related to attitudes, behaviors, self-image, and other important development issues for young people.

As you read the chapters that discussed these studies, you may have found yourself impressed by the findings, concerned about the outcomes, or wondering if there was other information available. Of course, a text of this nature is limited in the depth that can be provided, and as authors, we needed to be judicious in the studies we included. We attempted to include research that was methodologically sound, lacked apparent bias, and reported results that would be important for the reader.

But academic research has its limitations. Many of those limits are in methodology. Samples may not be truly representative of a given population. Effect sizes may be small. Statistical analyses may not be appropriate for the methods or may have limitations of their own. While the rigorous process of peer review is intended to prevent research studies from being published if they lack sufficient quality, each study has its limitations. We recognize that these critiques read as if they came directly from a textbook on research methodology.

What we believe is more important for the reader to consider is the nature of academic research and how it relates to the topic of youth consumption of SEIM. When an investigator has an idea for a research study, they develop one or more hypotheses (at least in the case of quantitative research; qualitative inquiry has its own limitations that are best discussed in a research text). The researcher develops a methodology to test the hypotheses, using statistical analyses. The analysis produces a result, and that result is considered significant if it meets certain criteria. When the results are statistically significant, the research is often published in an academic journal, and we see a result that reports, for example, that a correlation exists between adolescent consumption of SEIM and a lower age of first sexual encounters. This has importance, and we can point to the study as evidence that we should be attending to this issue when we work with adolescents.

But what is lacking in many academic journals are the studies that report that there were *no* significant results found. There are many reasons for this. Some journals are biased toward studies that prove their hypothesis; some academic would argue that most journals contain this bias. In other cases, an investigator may decide not to attempt to publish such a result, because of this bias or because the hypothesis was not proven. However, a lack of statistical significance proves something just as important, *that there is no (statistical) relationship between the two variables being observed.* So in the previous hypothetical research study, a lack of statistical significance would suggest that there is no relationship between SEIM consumption and the age of first sexual encounter.

But without seeing these results in the literature, we can have no idea as to how often this happens or what the implications are. Could it be the case that for every published study that suggests a relationship between SEIM consumption and some other variable, there are three studies that suggest there is no relationship? Would those findings be important to our work? We certainly think so, but we cannot know them because they are simply not available. In addition, there are studies that have found significant results suggesting a lack of relationship between some of the variables discussed throughout the text. We have included these where it was possible.

The other significant limitation in much of the academic research, as stated previously, is that there are very few studies that have found causation between variables. In other words, the research rarely states that consumption of SEIM *causes* any specific outcome but instead that they are correlated. Again, using the example of SEIM and age of sexual intercourse, a correlation only tells us that as SEIM consumption increases, the age of a first sexual encounter decreases. What we cannot know from this result is what caused the lower age of sexual activity. Are there other variables that were not part of the study that caused this result? Was it a constellation of different variables? Correlation does not equal causation, and we must be careful to remember this as we review the literature.

Rapid evolution: the technological boom

As discussed throughout this text, technology is constantly evolving. Recently, we have seen a more rapid evolution of technology than at any other time in history. As we alluded to at the opening of this text, many of us remember life without the Internet. We looked things up in encyclopedias. We went to libraries. We bought pornographic magazines and then later VHS tapes and DVDs at bookstores that catered exclusively to adults. Several decades ago, we all learned the buzzing and beeping sound of a computer modem that connected us to something called the World Wide Web, and if we were lucky, we heard that serotonin-releasing voice say, "You've got mail."

How times have changed. The Internet is accessible anytime, anywhere, with a pocket-sized computer that is exponentially more powerful than the large, clumsy desktop computers that made all of those beeping, buzzing sounds as they connected to the Internet. Televisions, video game systems, and refrigerators are all Internet-ready in today's limitless technological world. But this world does have limits that we do not even recognize because no one has yet broken those unknown barriers. This book will move from a laptop screen to a printing press, and in that time, someone might find a way to connect my garbage cans to the Internet, letting the trash collection company know it is time to stop by for a pick up.

As we discuss throughout the book, helping professionals need to stay abreast of technological advances if we are to be successful when working with digital natives. While digital immigrants will always retain some degree of a digital "accent," acclimation and assimilation can be helpful when we work with natives. To be successful, we must challenge ourselves to stay current with knowledge, even if we choose not to engage in the digital native's world. When we expect others to conform to our cultural norms, we run the risk of discounting theirs, which is antithetical to creating a healthy, effective, working alliance.

Understanding technology is very different from understanding a more static field, like psychological theory. Of course, new theories are developed and evolve over time, and anyone who practices those theories must stay abreast of those changes to be effective and ethical practitioners. But there is a qualitative difference when we consider technology. When we study the theories of Sigmund Freud, they are not going to change much from year to year, or even decade to decade. The Oedipus complex will be the same a year from now as it is today.

Technology, however, will most certainly not. As this book is being prepared to go to press, there is a popular social media application that allows people to take an image of their face and transform it so that the person appears decades older. It is a fun game to see what you or your friends might look like 20 years from now. The app is free, and on Monday of this week, it had taken the Internet by storm.

As we finalize the text, it is Thursday of the same week. It has been discovered that this app, that was wildly popular three days ago, is now the target of an investigation by the U.S. Congress (Bowman, 2019). It seems the app allows the developers access to all types of personal data, including the photos that are uploaded as well as other unconnected data, such as websites that the user has visited. It has also been discovered that the developers of the technology are based in St. Petersburg, Russia. This has raised concerns about how these data might be used by foreign governments to undermine elections in the United States and other countries. Also, given what we know about deepfake technology, concerns have been raised about how images may be used or manipulated.

That took four days.

Conclusion

This chapter provided a review and overview of many of the central issues discussed in this text, as well as context for how helping professionals can use the information here to better help adolescent clients as they navigate the world of Internet pornography. Examining issues related to attitudes, behaviors, self-image, culture, ethics, and law, this chapter provided helpers with the tools to make the most of this text. While there will always be more to write about pornography, technology, and the lives of young people, we hope this text provides a useful primer for those who want to help adolescents to live their best lives in a digital age.

Summary

- The impact of technology on the relationship between people from different generations has long been a challenge; in fact, it probably always has been.
- Cultural competence is developed through the development of our own knowledge, skill, and attitudes about the cultures other than our own, as well as the people who identify when them.

- Helping professionals must challenge themselves to consider their own values, beliefs, and attitudes about technology and the young people who live in a digital world.
- While research findings vary widely, and there is certainly ambiguity about what it all might mean for the helping practitioner, what we can glean from the findings is that when it comes to interventions, education is key.
- When we examine culture and pornography, issues such as age, gender, religion, worldview, political ideology, and sexual identity are crucial to the helping professional.
- Understanding the ethical and legal responsibilities of professional helpers is of the utmost importance for those who work with adolescents and issues of sexuality.
- Academic research has a number of limitations, including methodological concerns, issues related to causality, and bias in what is published in most academic journals.
- We have experienced a more rapid evolution of technology than at any other time in history; staying abreast of these, and future changes, is crucial to the helping professional.

References

American Counseling Association. (2014). *ACA code of ethics*. Alexandria, VA: Author.

Beggan, J. K., & Allison, S. T. (2003). "What sort of man reads playboy?" The self-reported influence of playboy on the construction of masculinity. *The Journal of Men's Studies*, *11*(2), 189–206. doi:10.3149/jms.1102.189

Bleakley, A., Hennessy, M., & Fishbein, M. (2011). A model of adolescents' seeking of sexual content in their media choices. *Journal of Sex Research*, *48*(4), 309–315. doi:10.1080/00224499.2010.497985

Bowman, E. (2019, July 17). Democrats issue warnings against viral Russia-based face-morphing app. *NPR*. Retrieved from www.npr.org/2019/07/17/742910309/democrats-issue-warnings-against-viral-russia-based-face-morphing-app

Häggström-Nordin, E., Sandberg, J., Hanson, U., & Tydén, T. (2006). "It's everywhere!" Young Swedish people's thoughts and reflections about pornography. *Scandinavian Journal of Caring Sciences*, *20*(4), 386–393. doi:10.1111/j.1471-6712.2006.00417.x

Hoffman, A. (2013). Bridging the digital divide: Using culture-infused counseling to enhance therapeutic work with digital youth. *Journal of Infant, Child, and Adolescent Psychotherapy*, *12*, 118–133. doi:10.1080/15289168.2013.791195

Perrin, P. C., Madanat, H. N., Barnes, M. D., Carolan, A., Clark, R. B., Ivins, N., & Tuttle, S. R. (2008). Health education's role in framing pornography as a public health issue: Local and national strategies with international implications. *Promotion & Education*, *15*, 11–18. doi:10.1177/1025382307088093

Perry, S. L. (2018). Not practicing what you preach: Religion and incongruence between pornography beliefs and usage. *Journal of Sex Research*, *55*(3), 369–380. doi:10.1080/00224499.2017.1333569

Perry, S. L., & Schleifer, C. (2017). Race and trends in pornography viewership, 1973–2016: Examining the moderating roles of gender and religion. *Journal of Sex Research*, *56*(1), 62–73. doi:10.1080/00224499.2017.1404959

Peter, J., & Valkenburg, P. (2009). Adolescents' exposure to sexually explicit Internet material and sexual satisfaction: A longitudinal study. *Human Communication Research*, *35*(2), 171–194. doi:10.1111/j.1468-2958.2009.01343.x

Prensky, M. (2001). Digital natives, digital immigrants. *On the Horizon*, *9*(6). Retrieved from www.marcprensky.com/writing/Prensky%20%20Digital%20Natives,%20Digital%20Immigrants%20-%20Part1.pdf

Rasmussen, K., & Bierman, A. (2016). How does religious attendance shape trajectories of pornography use across adolescence? *Journal of Adolescence*, *49*, 191–203. doi:10.1016/j.adolescence.2016.03.017

Ratts, M. J., Singh, A. A., Nassar-McMillan, S., Butler, S. K., & McCullough, J. R. (2016). Multicultural and social justice counseling competencies: Guidelines for the counseling profession. *Journal of Multicultural Counseling and Development*, *44*(1), 28–48. doi:10.1002/jmcd.12035

To, S., Kan, S., & Ngain, S. S. (2013). Interaction effects between exposure to explicit online materials and individual, family, and extramarital factors on Hong Kong high school students' beliefs about gender role equality and body-centered sexuality. *Youth and Society*, *47*, 747–768. doi:10.1177/0044118X13490764

Træen, B., Nilsen, T. S., & Stigum, H. (2006). Use of pornography in traditional media and on the internet in Norway. *Journal of Sex Research*, *43*(3), 245–254. doi:10.1080/00224490609552323

Tsaliki, L. (2011). Playing with porn: Greek children's explorations in pornography. *Sex Education*, *11*(3), 293–302. doi:10.1080/14681811.2011.590087

Tsitsika, A., Critselis, E., Kormas, G., Konstantoulaki, E., Constantopoulos, A., & Kafetzis, D. (2009). Adolescent pornographic Internet site use: A multivariate regression analysis of the predictive factors of use and psychosocial implications. *CyberPsychology & Behavior*, *12*(5), 545–550. doi:10.1089/cpb.2008.0346

Wallmyr, G., & Welin, C. (2006). Young people, pornography, and sexuality: Sources and attitudes. *The Journal of School Nursing*, *22*, 290–295. doi:10.1177/10598405060220050801

Index

ACA *Code of Ethics* (2014) 53, 75, 90, 121
academic research 122–123
addiction 49–51, 108
adolescence 1, 30, 52–53
adolescent: defined 5; development 3
amateur Internet pornography 63, 66
anal intercourse 48
anxiety 24–25
attitudes and beliefs 30–31, 42; addressing 39–42
attractiveness 66
autonomy 90

Baby Boomers 15, 119
behaviors, treating 54
beneficence 90
bias 4, 120; about adolescent sexuality 53–54; in academic journals 122; confirmation 108, 109, 120; in research 38, 39
blogging 23–24
body dissatisfaction 64; in the LGBTQ community 64–65
body dysmorphia 63
body esteem 37
body ideals 64, 69
body image 63–65; and sexual confidence 63, 68; *see also* physical attractiveness
body types 63–64, 66
breast size 67

casual sex 32, 47
causation 123
Centerfold Syndrome 31–32
child pornography 78, 93, 94–95; laws/statutes 94, 96, 112
Children's Internet Protection Act (CIPA) 105–106
child sexual abuse 97
cognitive-behavioral approaches 40, 54
cognitive dissonance 38, 80; *see also* dissonance
Communication Decency Act (CDA) 105
competence, boundaries of 91–92
compulsive behavior 3, 50
compulsive Internet use (CIU) 3
conduct issues/concerns 51, 54
confidentiality 90–91
confirmation bias 108, 109, 120
cultural competence 22, 23, 91–92, 119
cultural considerations in the helping process 81
cultural differences 22
cultural factors influencing SEIM consumption 120; age 75–76; gender 76–77; political ideology 77–78; religion 79–80; worldview 78–79
culture 8, 18, 21, 22, 39, 52, 101; and pornography 75, 120–121; *see also* cultural factors influencing SEIM consumption; popular culture
curiosity 55
cyberbullying 22
cybersex 3

Daniels, Stormy 21
deepfakes 109–110; legal recourse of victims 110–111
depression 24, 25, 50, 52, 80
DeVille, Cherie 21
Digital Economy Act 93, 106
digital immigrant 17, 18, 119, 123
digital native 17–18, 79, 119, 123; and the helping relationship 21–25; subgenerations of 18
dissonance 30, 36, 38; *see also* cognitive dissonance

ectomorphs 61
education *see* sexual education
endomorphs 61
ethical codes 89–90; and laws 92
ethical decision-making 98–101
ethical responsibility to youth 90–91
ethics 89, 121
European Convention on Human Rights (ECHR) 106

Facebook 24
false light statutes 111
fidelity 90
First Amendment 105, 106, 111
free speech and expression 93, 105–106; and deepfakes 111

gender-stereotypical sexual beliefs 34–36
generational differences 14, 17, 119
generations 14; defined 15
Generation X 15, 119
Generation Z 15; characteristics of 16; and technology 16–17
genital esteem 37
genitalia 66

"hardcore" pornography 94
heteronormative bias 53
high-risk behavior 48–49

informed consent 91, 92
Institutional Review boards 92
Internet 2; accessibility of 6; adolescent use statistics 3; defined 6; and pornography 2, 21; problematic use 23; *see also* Internet pornography
Internet pornography 3, 49–50, 61, 62, 75; addiction to 49–51; amateur 63, 66; and body image 63–65; laws related to 93–95; legal and ethical issues 88–89; and physical attractiveness 66; and religion 79–80; and self-esteem 68; and sexual-related body parts 66–68; *see also* SEIM consumption; sexually explicit Internet material (SEIM)
intervention, approaches to 54–55

Jameson, Jenna 21
justice 90

law: and advancements in technology 95–96; and ethics 121

laws 92–93; and legal issues/obligations 92–97; related to Internet pornography 93–95
legal arguments 93
LGBTQA+ community 53
LGBTQ community, body dissatisfaction in 64–65
LGBTQ youth, and SEIM 81–82
loneliness 23

mandated reporting 91, 96, 97
masculinity validation 31
media: and attitudes towards gender 35; and heterosexual male sexuality 31; sexual/sexualized 19, 32, 37; sexually suggestive 21; *see also* popular culture
mesomorphs 61–62
Millennials 15, 18; characteristics of 16; and technology 15–16, 17
Miller test 94
Miller v. California 93
morality 77, 78, 79, 89, 108
moral principles 90, 121
music 19–20
music videos 19–20

National Center on Sexual Exploitation (NCSE) 107, 108
negativity bias 53
net neutrality 106
news 20–21
nonmaleficence 90
nonrelational sex 31
non-Western cultures 78, 79

objectification 31, 34, 63, 68; *see also* sexual object
obscene pornography 94
Obscene Publications Act 94
obscenity 93–94
obscenity laws 94
obsessions 50
oral sex 47

parent-adolescent interactions 41
peer interactions 41
penis size 62, 67
permissive sexual attitudes 32–33, 39
Personal Sexual Norms Scale 32
personal values/beliefs 91, 121
physical attractiveness 66
political ideology 77–78
polyvictimization 49

popular culture 19, 21; deepfake videos 110; music 19–20; news 20–21; television 20
pornographic Internet sites, defined 6
pornography: definitions of 5–6, 52; degrading portrayal of females 36; Internet and 2, 21; intersection of culture and 120–121; as a public health issue 106–107; *see also* Internet pornography; sexually explicit Internet material (SEIM)
Pornography: A Public Health Crisis 107
positive technology 24
progressive sexual attitudes 32, 33
psychoeducation 41, 42, 55, 120; and sexting 112–113
public health issue 106–107

rape 108
religion/religious beliefs 51, 79–80, 121
Reno v. ACLU 105
research: academic 122–123; bias in 38, 39; with youth participants 92
resolutions 107
revenge porn 96, 112; laws 111

same-sex SEIM 81–82
SEIM consumption: addiction 49–51; and age 75–76; and body dissatisfaction 64; and causality 52; and Centerfold Syndrome 31–32; and conduct issues 51; and gender 76–77; and gender-stereotypical sexual beliefs 34–36; and high-risk behavior 48–49; and mental health concerns 52; as a normative experience 39; and objectification 31, 36; and onset of sexual activity 47–48; and participation in sexual activity 47; and peer interactions 41; and permissive sexual attitudes 32–33; and political ideology 77–78; positive associations with 68–69; prevalence of 7–8; and progressive sexual attitudes 33; and religion 79–80; and sexual aggression 49; and sexual norms 32; and sexual self-development 36–38; and substance abuse 52; unintentional 7, 52, 76; and worldview 78–79
SEIM consumption studies, limitations and considerations 38–39, 121–122
self-esteem 36, 62, 65, 68–69
self-image 62–63, 67; reflections on 65; *see also* body image

self-reporting 8
sexting 96, 111–114
sexual aggression 49, 109; *see also* sexual violence
sexual assault 49
sexual attitudes 32–33
sexual education 40–41, 55, 119–120; SEIM as a form of 54–55
sexual esteem 37
sexual expression 34, 93
sexual harassment 49
sexually explicit Internet material (SEIM) 1, 2, 21; addiction to 49–51; adolescents and 2–3; and attitudes and beliefs about sexual relationships 30; and body image 62–65; defined 5; focus on specific body parts in 67; government involvement in 105–108; perceived realism of 32–33, 37; prevalence of adolescent consumption 7–8; same-sex 81; as sexual education 54–55; and unrealistic expectations 61; violent 49; *see also* SEIM consumption
sexually explicit material *see* pornography
sexual norms 32
sexual object 34, 35, 36, 40; *see also* objectification
sexual preoccupancy 37–38
sexual reductionism 31
sexual satisfaction 37
sexual self-development 36–38
sexual violence 20, 49, 108
smartphone 16, 96
social learning theory 19
social media 3, 21, 22, 97; and deepfakes 110; as a screening tool 24; and sexting 112; sexually explicit 47
stereotypical gender attitudes and beliefs 34–36
substance abuse 52, 54

technological advances 123–124; and the law 95–96
technology 14, 16–17; attitudes and beliefs about 22–23; as a cultural construct 118–119; rapid evolution of 123–124; related to wellness and counseling 24–25
technology-assisted self-help interventions 24–25
technology-based sexual harassment 49
TechnoWellness 24
TechnoWellness Inventory (TWI) 24
television 20

terminology 5–6
therapeutic relationship, impact of technology on 21–22
trauma-informed techniques and theories 54
trophyism 31

Universal Declaration of Human Rights 106

unrealistic sexual expectations and standards 61
unsafe sex 53

veracity 90
victimization 49
voyeurism 31

Western cultures 78, 79

Printed in Great Britain
by Amazon